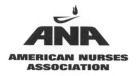

AMERICAN NURSES ASSOCIATION

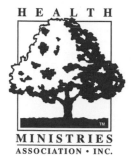

HEALTH

MINISTRIES
ASSOCIATION • INC.

Scope AND
Standards
OF PRACTICE

Faith Community Nursing

2ND EDITION

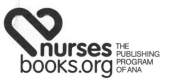

nurses THE
books.org PUBLISHING
PROGRAM
OF ANA

American Nurses Association
Silver Spring, Maryland
2012

Library of Congress Cataloging-in-Publication Data

Faith community nursing : scope and standards of practice. — 2nd ed.
  p. ; cm.

Rev. ed. of: Faith community nursing / Health Ministries Association. 2005.

Includes bibliographical references and index.

Summary: "Delineates the practice of faith community nurses, which integrates the health and care of body, mind, and spirit in the context of a faith community, its professional roles, activities, expected accountabilities and competency levels per RN knowledge, skills, abilities, and judgment, education, professional development, and the specialty's history/legacy and trends"—Provided by publisher.

ISBN 978-1-55810-429-7—ISBN 978-1-55810-430-3 (pdf eBook)—ISBN 978-1-55810-433-4 (pdf eBook for site licenses)—ISBN 978-1-55810-431-0 (eBook, Mobipocket format)

I. American Nurses Association. II. Health Ministries Association. Faith community nursing.
[DNLM: 1. Community Health Nursing—standards—Practice Guideline. 2. Spirituality—Practice Guideline. 3. Holistic Nursing--standards—Practice Guideline. 4. Nursing Process—standards—Practice Guideline. WY 87]

610.73'43—dc23

2011047488

Health Ministries Association (HMA) and American Nurses Association (ANA) are national professional associations. This joint HMA–ANA publication (*Faith Community Nursing: Scope and Standards of Practice, Second Edition*) reflects the thinking of the faith community nursing specialty on various issues and should be reviewed in conjunction with state board of nursing policies and practices. State law, rules, and regulations govern the practice of nursing, while *Faith Community Nursing: Scope and Standards of Practice, Second Edition* guides faith community nurses in the application of their professional skills and responsibilities.

ISBN-13: 978-1-55810-429-7   SAN: 851-3481   5K   01/2012

First printing: January 2012

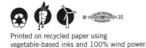

Printed on recycled paper using
vegetable-based inks and 100% wind power.

Contents

Contributors

Faith Community Nursing Scope and Standards of Practice Work Group

Alyson J. Breisch, MSN, RN, FCN

Proprietor, Breisch Health Education, PLLC, Durham, North Carolina; Chair, Health Ministries Association FCN Standards Work Group, 2011

Ms. Breisch has more than 40 years experience in nursing administration, academic education, and advanced practice nursing as a clinical nurse specialist and adult nurse practitioner. She directed the graduate degree program in Health and Nursing Ministries of Duke Divinity School and Duke University School of Nursing and developed a continuing education curriculum for faith community nursing. She has been a faith community nurse for 12 years and a Commissioned Minister of Congregational Health for 5 years. Ms. Breisch is active in several professional nursing organizations. She is Director of Practice and Education on the Board of Directors of Health Ministries Association.

Jean Bokinskie, PhD, RN, FCN

Associate Professor of Nursing and Director of the Parish Nurse Ministry Program, Concordia College, Moorhead, Minnesota

Dr. Bokinskie has taught in nursing education for more than 20 years and has served as an administrator in faith community nursing for 10 years. Her dissertation study was focused on parish nursing education, administration, and practice. She has published articles on parish nursing practice, completed a number of research studies on parish nursing practice and outcomes, and provided numerous presentations on faith community nursing. She is active in several professional organizations.

Katora P. Campbell, DrPHc, MSN, RN, CHES
Parish Nurse Manager, Parish Nurse Program, Midlands Partnership for Community Health, Columbia, South Carolina
Dr. Campbell supervises the work of parish nurses serving 19 churches, including the oversight of parish nurse services for low-income senior apartments. In 2001, she received the Excellence in Nursing Award from Sigma Theta Tau at Clemson University for her pioneering work in parish nursing. She is currently completing a doctorate degree in health services policy and management from the University of South Carolina.

Sheila Carroll, MSN, RN, APRN-C, FCN
Director, Rose Garden Center for Hope and Healing, Covington, Kentucky
With a varied nursing career Ms. Carroll changed direction upon graduation as a family nurse practitioner in 1995 from the University of Kentucky. Experience in family practice and emergency medicine led her to another phase of nursing. In October 2009, in cooperation with St. Elizabeth Healthcare in Covington, Kentucky, the Rose Garden Center for Hope and Healing was begun to serve the medically indigent in the Northern Kentucky area. What began as a health ministry continues as the Center grows into a team of an all-volunteer staff in a free clinic led by faith.

Nancy L. Rago Durbin, MS, RN, FCN
Director, Parish Nurse Ministry and Parish Nurse Support Network, Advocate Health Care, Park Ridge, Illinois
With more than 22 years of experience in health ministry, Ms. Durbin has been a leader in developing resources for faith community nursing that include policies, procedures, competencies, program evaluation, and data measurement. She is active in several professional organizations, including Health Ministries Association, and is currently chair of the Faith Community Nurse Recognition Task Force, which works with the American Nurses Credentialing Center and Health Ministries Association to develop a certification process for the specialty practice of faith community nursing.

Marlene Feagan, MA, BSN, RN, FCN
Health Ministries Coordinator, St. Elizabeth Healthcare, Northern Kentucky
For more than 15 years, Ms. Feagan has worked as a health ministries and faith community nursing coordinator. She developed, implemented, and manages a wholistic wellness and prevention model of care for faith

communities and the community at large. She also developed a unique wholistic-based geriatric care management model. She is active in several professional organizations and holds leadership positions for the Health Ministries Association. She has presented and written on health ministries, faith community nursing, spirituality in nursing, and aging issues locally, regionally, and nationally.

Paulette Golden, MS, RN, FCN
Manager, Community Health and Faith Community Nursing Programs, Texas Health Harris Methodist Hospital, Fort Worth, Texas

With more than 30 years nursing experience in a variety of settings of critical care, occupational health, education, and community health, Ms. Golden has worked in the area of faith community nursing for the past nine years. She is active in several professional organizations, including leadership positions in the Texas State Health Ministries Association and the Parish Nurse Faculty through the International Parish Nurse Resources Center.

Beverly Lunsford, PhD, CNS-BC, RN
Associate Research Professor, School of Nursing, The George Washington University, Washington, D.C.

Dr. Lunsford has more than 35 years experience in nursing practice, education, administration, and research. She has taught nursing courses, including research, theory, population health, spirituality and health, and palliative care nursing. Dr. Lunsford has developed new programs for wholistic adolescent and young adult health care and palliative care. She writes grants to fund research and healthcare programs, especially to improve health care for underserved, vulnerable, and disenfranchised populations. She currently directs two grant-funded research projects in geriatric education.

Vickie L. Morley, MSN, RN, FCN
Faith Community Nurse Coordinator, Shenandoah University, Winchester, Virginia

Mrs. Morley has 30 years of nursing experience in a variety of practice settings. Specialty practices include pediatrics, faith community nursing, academia, and continuing education. She has a wealth of experience in faith community nursing as an educator and practitioner. As a national speaker, advocate, and educator, Mrs. Morley is passionate about promoting the specialty practice of faith community nursing.

Katia Reinert, MSN, CRNP, FCN-BC, PHCNS-BC
Family Nurse Practitioner, Smith Ho Internal Medicine; Health Ministries Director, Seventh-Day Adventist Church in North America, Silver Spring, Maryland
Prior to accepting the call to serve in her current role, Ms. Reinert served in the nursing profession at Washington Adventist Hospital for 15 years as a critical care nurse, occupational health nurse practitioner, Faith Community Nursing Coordinator, and Health Ministry Clinical Supervisor for Adventist HealthCare. She fostered medical–religious partnerships and coordinated faith community nursing and lay health ministry training for health professionals and lay ministers. She is currently pursuing doctoral studies in the area of religion and health.

Marilyn Seiler, MS, RN, FCN
Parish Nurse Coordinator, Catholic Parish of St. John the Baptist, Edmond, Oklahoma, and Catholic Parishes of Stillwater, Oklahoma
While serving as the Parish Nurse Coordinator for three Catholic parishes, Ms. Seiler has also been active in providing foundation and ongoing education for faith community nurses in Oklahoma. She has 27 years experience in all types and all positions of home care agencies. In addition, she was a home health consultant with an emphasis in documentation, quality, and general administrative issues. She has authored publications related to home health and faith community nursing.

Roberta Schweitzer, PhD, RN, FCN
Assistant Professor, School of Nursing, College of Health and Human Science, Purdue University, West Lafayette, Indiana; Education Director, Greater Lafayette Parish Nurse Development Center, Lafayette, Indiana
Dr. Schweitzer's 35 years of nursing experience include advanced practice, academic education, and research. For 20 years, she has been involved in the development of faith community nursing practice. Dr. Schweitzer served on the editorial staff for three editions of the International Parish Nurse Resource Center's Foundations of Faith Community Nursing curriculum. Currently, Dr. Schweitzer's faith community nursing practice and education guide her research trajectory as well as her data-based, peer-reviewed publications in nursing journals which focus on spiritual leadership in faith community nursing, spiritual well-being, and health-related quality of life in coping with chronic illness.

Angela Sheehan, MS, RN, FCN
Director, Faith Community/Parish Nurse Program, Seton Health, Troy, New York
As a nurse working for 37 years in many settings, Ms. Sheehan's primary focus in care delivery has become spirituality in nursing. After obtaining a CNS in mental health, she completed coursework for Nurse Practitioner in mental health in 2007. She is dedicated to faith community nursing and believes that mental health and spirituality need to be better integrated, as well as the physical aspects, for a truly holistic healthcare model. Ms. Sheehan believes the art of nursing can be actualized through faith community nursing and works tirelessly to integrate spirituality in all that nurses do.

Norma R. Small, PhD, APRN
Historian, Health Ministries Association, Arnold, Maryland
Dr. Small has more than 50 years experience in nursing practice, education, and administration. She was a founding member of the Health Ministries Association (HMA) and was HMA's consultant for obtaining the American Nurses Association's recognition of parish nursing as a specialty. She was involved in the first publication of *Scope and Standards of Parish Nursing Practice* (HMA, 1998). In 1990, she started the first graduate program in parish health nursing at Georgetown University. Dr. Small currently consults and lectures in the areas of health ministry and faith community nursing.

Sharon Stanton, MS, RN, FCN
Coordinator, Center for Health Ministries, Catholic Healthcare West–Arizona, Chandler, Arizona
Specializing in leadership development, Ms. Stanton has almost 50 years of experience. She has worked in multiple diverse roles integrating public health, migrant health, home health, and academia. Ms. Stanton has worked in the field of faith health ministry for more than 16 years developing best-practice models in the Southeast and Southwest. She currently coordinates and oversees Catholic Healthcare West–Arizona's replicable model for faith health ministry, a collaboration between two major hospitals and 19 faith communities. The model integrates faith community nursing into the total patient care team, provides continuity of care, and increases the potential for data retrieval and research. Ms. Stanton is a cojourner of the Sisters of Saint Francis.

Chris VanDenburgh, MSN, RN, FCN
Coordinator, Faith Community Nursing and Health Ministry, Kettering Health Network, Kettering, Ohio
In addition to faith community nursing, Ms. VanDenburgh's areas of training include clinical pastoral education and critical incident stress management. She has been involved in faith community nursing for many years, both as a full-time, paid faith community nurse and as an educator and program coordinator. Ms. VanDenburgh serves as the Director of Health Ministry for her denominational organization and has been a speaker and presenter on spiritual care, spirituality and healing, and faith community nursing both in the United States and abroad.

Denise Viker, BSN, RN, FCN
Director of Congregational Health Services, Duet, Phoenix, Arizona
Ms. Viker has more than 25 years of experience teaching and managing nurses in a variety of nursing specialties. She has served as a faith community nurse at Desert Cross Lutheran Church in Tempe, Arizona, for more than 10 years. She applies this experience in her role as director by educating and supporting a network of faith community nurses throughout the state of Arizona. She is working collaboratively with students from Arizona State University to develop a faith community nursing database.

Susan Ward, PhD, RN
Nursing Professor, Nebraska Methodist College, Josie Harper Campus, Omaha, Nebraska
Dr. Ward has been an educator for 21 years in undergraduate and graduate nursing programs at Nebraska Methodist College. She has been instrumental at the local, regional, and national levels in moving faith community nursing practice forward. She served as a faith community nurse at Countryside Community Church in Omaha, Nebraska. Her work includes presenting at conferences related to spirituality and health, editing the International Parish Nurse Resource Center (IPNRC) curriculum and foundational documents for global Parish Nurse Resource Centers in conjunction with the IPNRC, and serving on the work group for the 2005 edition of *Faith Community Nursing: Scope and Standards of Practice.* She has presented at professional engagements and taught Nebraska Methodist College's online parish nursing course for more than 10 years.

Andrea M. West, PhD, RN, FCN

Director of Curriculum and Research, International Parish Nurse Resource Center, St. Louis, Missouri

Dr. West has more than 25 years experience in nursing education at the diploma, baccalaureate, and graduate levels, including serving as dean of a baccalaureate program. She has served on a variety of nursing and university committees and has been active in the American Nurses Association through the Oklahoma Nurses Association, in the National League for Nursing through the Oklahoma League for Nursing, and in Sigma Theta Tau. Her community activities include membership on a regional hospital board and a three-level care community for the elderly. She coordinated the education program for faith community nursing in Oklahoma.

Paula White, BSN, MSA, RN, FCN

Faith Community Nursing Coordinator, Borgess Health, Kalamazoo, Michigan

With more than 40 years of varied nursing experience across the continuum of care, Ms. White has been active in parish nursing since 1991. Since 2004, she has coordinated Borgess Health's outreach to assist nurses in beginning and sustaining congregational health ministries in nine counties of southwest Michigan. She is a member of the American Nurses Association, Sigma Theta Tau, and the Health Ministries Association. She is an active member of the International Parish Nurse Resource Center faculty, teaching the foundations of faith community nursing, and is a founding member and the treasurer of the West Michigan Partners in Health Ministry.

Diana Williams, MSN, RN, FCN

Director, Community Resources, Our Lady of Bellefonte Hospital, Bon Secours Kentucky Health System, Ashland, Kentucky

Under Ms. Williams's leadership, Our Lady of Bellefonte Hospital was the first organization in its service area to offer health ministry–faith community nursing to local congregations. Since its inception in the fall of 1996, the ministry has developed partnerships with approximately 50 congregations. Ms. Williams is a fellow of the Kentucky Public Health Leadership Institute and the Bon Secours Ministry Leadership Formation Intensive. She is a member of both the Bon Secours and the Kentucky Parish Nurse Networks.

Deborah Ziebarth, MSN, RN, FCN
Assistant Professor of Nursing, Herzing University, Brookfield Campus, Milwaukee, Wisconsin

With more than 30 years of experience in nursing, Ms. Ziebarth has worked extensively in the areas of community health, global health, and academic education. She received national recognition for her management of community-based nursing programs (the American Hospital Association's 2006 Nova Award and the Volunteer Hospital Association's 2008 Best in Class Award). She was recognized in 2010 by Wisconsin Nursing Association with a Face of Nursing Award and recently published the Wisconsin Parish Nurse Minimum Educational Standards, which includes her research. Active on the Wisconsin Parish Nurse Coalition Board, she has held the position of education chair since 2003. She has consulted with the International Parish Nurse Resource Center on various projects. Recently, Ms. Ziebarth joined Herzing University as a member of the nursing faculty.

ANA Staff

Carol Bickford, PhD, RN-BC, CPHIMS – Content editor
Yvonne Daley Humes, MSA – Project coordinator
Maureen E. Cones, Esq. – Legal counsel
Eric Wurzbacher –Project editor
Melaney Johnson –Printing and manufacturing coordinator

About the American Nurses Association

The American Nurses Association (ANA) is the only full-service professional organization representing the interests of the nation's 3.1 million registered nurses through its constituent/state nurses associations and its organizational affiliates. The ANA advances the nursing profession by fostering high standards of nursing practice, promoting the rights of nurses in the workplace, projecting a positive and realistic view of nursing, and lobbying the Congress and regulatory agencies on healthcare issues affecting nurses and the public. More at www.NursingWorld.org.

About Health Ministries Association, Inc.

Health Ministries Association, Inc. (HMA), a nonprofit membership organization, is a support network for people of faith who promote whole-person health through faith groups in the communities they serve. HMA is the recognized professional membership organization for the nursing specialty of faith community nursing and promotes education, research utilization, and evidence-based practice. By providing information, guidelines, and resources, HMA assists and encourages individuals, families, and communities as they develop whole-person health programs, utilize community resources, and educate others on the interdependent health of body, mind, and spirit. More at www.hmassoc.org/.

About Nursesbooks.org, The Publishing Program of ANA

Nursesbooks.org publishes books on ANA core issues and programs, including ethics, leadership, quality, specialty practice, advanced practice, and the profession's enduring legacy. Best known for the foundational documents of the profession on ethics, scope and standards of practice, and social policy, Nursesbooks.org is the publisher for the professional, career-oriented nurse, reaching and serving nurse educators, administrators, managers, and researchers, as well as staff nurses in the course of their professional development. More at www.Nursesbooks.org/.

Introduction

The American Nurses Association (ANA) published the first *Scope and Standards of Parish Nursing Practice* in 1998. As the practice of parish nursing evolved, the title of the specialty practice was changed to *faith community nursing* with the publication of *Faith Community Nursing: Scope and Standards of Practice* in 2005. Since then, there have been dramatic changes in health care as well as the nursing profession. *Faith Community Nursing: Scope and Standards of Practice, Second Edition*, describes the specialty practice of faith community nursing for the nursing profession, faith community nurses, other healthcare providers, spiritual leaders, employers, insurers, healthcare consumers, families, and members of faith communities. The unique scope of knowledge and the standards of practice and professional performance for a faith community nurse (FCN) are discussed.

Function of the Scope of Practice Statement of Faith Community Nursing

The scope of practice statement describes the *who, what, where, when, why,* and *how* of the practice of faith community nursing. The answers to these questions provide a complete picture of the practice, its boundaries, and its membership. *Nursing: Scope and Standards of Practice, Second Edition* (ANA, 2010a) applies to all professional registered nurses engaged in practice, regardless of specialty, practice setting, or educational preparation. With *Code of Ethics for Nurses with Interpretive Statements* (ANA, 2001) and *Nursing's Social Policy Statement: The Essence of the Profession* (ANA, 2010b), it forms the foundation of practice for all registered nurses. The scope of faith community nursing practice is specific to this specialty but builds on the scope of practice expected of all registered nurses.

Function of the Standards of Faith Community Nursing Practice

Standards are "authoritative statements defined and promoted by the profession by which the quality of practice, service, or education can be evaluated" (ANA, 2010a, p. 67). Standards reflect the values and priorities of the profession and provide direction for professional nursing practice and a framework for evaluation of this practice. The standards of faith community nursing practice are specific to this specialty but build on the standards of professional nursing practice applicable to all registered nurses.

Development of *Faith Community Nursing: Scope and Standards of Practice, Second Edition*

Health Ministries Association (HMA), the professional membership organization for nurses in this specialty, and ANA collaborated in the development and publication of *Faith Community Nursing: Scope and Standards of Practice* in 2005. With the publication of *Nursing: Scope and Standards of Practice, Second Edition* (ANA, 2010a), all specialty scope and standards of practice are now being revised. For continuity and consistency, that publication was used as the template when developing this new edition.

Following the 2005 revision, the HMA board requested volunteers to serve on a working group to review and revise the scope and standards for faith community nursing. Twenty-one practicing nurses representing different areas of the country and various roles in this specialty practice contributed to this revision. A draft copy of the document was posted on the HMA web site for public review. Responses were received and carefully considered in creating the final document. As a result, this document provides a national perspective on the current practice of this specialty of faith community nursing.

Summary

The scope and standards of practice for faith community nursing reflect the commitment of the Health Ministries Association to work with the American Nurses Association to promote an understanding of faith community nursing as a specialized practice in the interprofessional practice arena of diverse faith communities. HMA is the national professional organization representing faith community nurses and others working in the expanding faith community arena.

As the diversity of participating faith communities expands in rural areas, towns, and cities, the difficulty in finding all-inclusive terminology to describe the beliefs and practices that have evolved from the variety of traditions becomes more apparent. Terms used in this document indicate an effort to include many faith traditions and not to promote any one particular faith tradition.

Faith Community Nursing: Scope and Standards of Practice, Second Edition, reflects current faith community nursing practice from a national perspective, the professional and ethical standards of the nursing profession, and the legal scope and standards of professional nursing practice. They are dynamic and subject to testing and change.

Scope of Faith Community Nursing Practice

Definition and Overview of Faith Community Nursing

Faith community nursing is a specialized practice of professional nursing that focuses on the intentional care of the spirit as well as on the promotion of wholistic health and prevention or minimization of illness within the context of a faith community.

The term *faith community nurse* (FCN) is used to represent a registered nurse specializing in faith community nursing. The FCN is knowledgeable in two primary areas—professional nursing and spiritual care. The faith community nurse provides spiritual care in the faith community as well as in the broader community. The goals of an FCN are the protection, promotion, and optimization of health and abilities; the prevention of illness and injury; and the alleviation of suffering in the context of the values, beliefs, and practices of a faith community, such as a church, congregation, parish, synagogue, temple, mosque, or faith-based community agency.

Healthcare consumer is the term used by the American Nurses Association to define a person, client, family, group, community, or population that is the focus of attention and to which the registered nurse is providing services as sanctioned by the state regulatory bodies. In narratives within the specialty of faith community nursing, other terms such as *parishioner*, *congregant*, or *faith community member* may also be included as descriptive terms. The term *healthcare consumer* may refer to the faith community as a whole, or to groups, families, and individuals in the faith community. People from the broader community may also seek the services of the FCN.

The FCN uses the nursing process to address the spiritual, physical, mental, and social health of the healthcare consumer. With an intentional focus on spiritual health, the FCN primarily uses the interventions of education, counseling, prayer, presence, active listening, advocacy, referral, and a wide variety of resources available to the faith community. The faith community nurse may also train and supervise volunteers from the faith community. As an actively licensed registered nurse, the FCN provides nursing care based on standards and professional experience, legal expectations, and education. The FCN focuses on the needs of the healthcare consumer population and the position as defined by the faith community. The FCN collaborates with other specialties, such as primary care, community health, hospice, rehabilitation, home health, acute care, critical care, integrative health, and long-term care in other aspects of care for the faith community and its members.

This document—in conjunction with *Nursing's Social Policy Statement: The Essence of the Profession* (ANA, 2010b), *Nursing: Scope and Standards of Practice, Second Edition* (ANA, 2010a), and *Code of Ethics for Nurses with Interpretive Statements* (ANA, 2001)—delineates the professional responsibilities of an FCN. FCNs are also bound by the laws, statutes, and regulations related to nursing practice for their state, commonwealth, or territory.

Evolution of Faith Community Nursing

Nursing has its historical foundation deeply rooted in faith and health, as well as in the ancient and recent traditions of many religions. Faith traditions established rules for public health, including care of persons with infectious diseases. These communities also included visiting the sick and caring for infants and the elderly as religious duty. This sense of duty to care for a community's members expanded to include "care for the stranger" and was the basis for early *diakonas*—houses for strangers—which became the first charity hospitals. In the 12th, 13th, and 14th centuries, a new cadre of men serving in nursing orders emerged and provided care to men and women wounded in wars and to lepers. Religious orders also provided care for persons with mental illnesses. During the 16th century, more than 100 female religious orders were founded specifically to do nursing.

The faith and health link evolved over time and has been influenced by cultural, political, social, and economic events. Religious groups founded hospitals to provide care to vulnerable populations, such as the poor, immigrant, and homeless. In the late 1800s churches began to reclaim their role in healing. Diaconal ministries that developed in Europe migrated to the United States, and immigrant churches imported the work of deaconesses and other religious orders to provide health care to those in their communities. These religious affiliations were instrumental in developing schools of nursing during the 20th century.

Florence Nightingale, trained through the Deaconess Institution in Kaiserswerth, Germany, felt called to the service of the sick. In addition to her nursing education, she was a theological scholar and writer. Her religious philosophy and belief in a higher power was the foundation for her work to promote nursing as a trained profession, establish a public healthcare system that included health promotion and preventive medicine, and advocate for health issues as a social activist. The rich history of nursing's evolution is exquisitely collected in Patricia Donahue's (1996) *Nursing, The Finest Art: An Illustrated History*.

In the late 1950s, Halbert Dunn, a physician, developed a public health concept that he called high-level wellness. His writings were a catalyst for wellness centers that began in the 1970s. A growing public interest in complementary and alternative medicine influenced Western conventional medical care to incorporate aspects of these models into integrated care. This growing interest and focus on health promotion and wellness influenced the development of faith community nursing.

In 1979, Rev. Dr. Granger Westberg created wholistic health centers in Christian congregations, staffed by a treatment/healing team, comprising a doctor, a nurse, a social worker, and a pastoral counselor. The nurses in these centers were referred to as "parish nurses." Since then various other faith communities have established programs of health and healing led by a registered nurse. The word "parish" in *parish nurse* is not appropriate in all faith traditions, so faith communities have created different titles for this specialized nursing role. To have one name inclusive of all faith traditions and to accurately label the location and focus of practice, the specialty practice described in this document is *faith community nursing*. In a given setting, the faith community nurse may be referred to as a *parish nurse, congregational nurse, health ministry nurse, crescent nurse*, or *health and wellness nurse*.

Westberg used the term *wholistic health* to define a whole or completely integrated approach to health and health care that integrates the physical and spiritual aspects of the whole person. The principles of wholistic health arose from the understanding that human beings strive for wholeness in their relationship to their God or higher power, themselves, their families, the society, and the environment in which they live. Based on its historic meaning, *wholistic* is the preferred spelling when referring to the health care provided by faith community nurses.

Nurse-led programs within and beyond Judeo-Christian faith communities continue to grow and evolve. The common expectation across faith traditions is that the professional registered nurse functioning as an FCN possesses a depth of understanding of the faith community's traditions, as well as competence as a registered nurse, using the nursing process so that the nursing care integrates care of the spirit with care of the body and mind.

Assumptions of Faith Community Nursing

These five assumptions underlie faith community nursing:

- Health and illness are human experiences.

- Health is the integration of the spiritual, physical, psychological, and social aspects of the healthcare consumer to create a sense of harmony with self, others, the environment, and a higher power.

- Health may be experienced in the presence of disease or injury.

- The presence of illness does not preclude health nor does optimal health preclude illness.

- Healing is the process of integrating the body, mind, and spirit to create wholeness, health, and a sense of well-being, even when the healthcare consumer's illness is not cured.

Focusing on Spiritual Care in Nursing

Nurses have long observed that when illness or brokenness occurs, healthcare consumers—whether individually or with their family or friends—may turn to their source of spiritual strength for reassurance, support, and healing. *Nursing: Scope and Standards of Practice, Second Edition* (ANA, 2010a) reaffirms that spiritual care is a part of all nursing practice. The primary focus of the FCN is the intentional care of the spirit, differentiating this specialty practice from the general practice of a registered nurse. Within this specialized knowledge base, each FCN will demonstrate competence on a continuum of expertise.

A variety of tools for spiritual assessment have been developed and tested for reliability and validity. These tools, varying from simple screening to in-depth assessments, are increasingly used in nursing practice. Because, in general, the use of spiritual assessment tools has not been taught to providers from other disciplines, the FCN may provide leadership to the staff in the selection and application of assessment tools.

After analyzing the assessment data, the FCN selects the diagnoses to describe actual or potential needs of the healthcare consumer, including spiritual needs. These diagnoses then provide the basis for interventions to achieve the outcomes for which the nurse is accountable.

Treatment may or may not cure an affliction. However, it is still possible through care of the spirit for a person to be healed even if a cure—physical restoration—does not occur. A person may be dying from cancer, but if a broken relationship between family members has been reconciled or the person is at peace with the circumstances, this may be considered healing.

Assault, betrayal, accident, or death of a member of the community can affect an entire faith community. Members of all ages may manifest anger, grief, depression, anxiety, fear, and spiritual or physical pain in varying degrees. An FCN's response to such an event is complex. Beyond identifying and meeting the needs of individuals and families, the FCN treats the whole-faith community as a healthcare consumer. Assessment focuses on identifying the educational and supportive needs of the whole-faith community. Interventions occur at three different levels: community, family or group, and individual.

The FCN will address a variety of issues that threaten the wholistic health of persons in the faith community:

- Individuals or families may lack food, shelter, transportation, income, or health care.

- Victims of violence, abuse, or exploitation in a variety of settings, including domestic settings, may seek solace or sanctuary.

- Adult children of aging parents may seek guidance in talking with or determining the appropriate living situation for a parent, and ongoing assistance from the faith community.

- Victims of natural disasters and other life-altering emergencies may require various forms of assistance.

To respond to these and other situations wholistically, an FCN draws on professional skills that integrate spiritual care and nursing care, as well as the resources of individuals and groups both within and beyond the faith community, to provide a wholistic response. Some healthcare consumers will require support of basic needs so that they have the time and space to reflect on spiritual issues; for others, spiritual care will be the direct response. The form of spiritual care will depend on the beliefs and practices of the faith community; the desire of the faith community, the group, or the individual; the skills of the FCN; and the collaboration of other staff members and volunteers.

Health Advocacy and Faith Community Nursing

One of the key aspects of faith community nursing is health advocacy. As stated in *Code of Ethics for Nurses with Interpretive Statements* (ANA, 2001, p. 16), the faith community nurse "promotes, advocates for, and strives to protect the health, safety, and rights of the patient." In the settings for faith community nursing, this often includes advocating for appropriate levels of care for vulnerable populations and those with limited access to healthcare resources. Such advocacy may include initiating referrals for clinical treatment, obtaining home care resources, or assisting with extended care arrangements. Faith community nurses may promote advocacy for healthcare consumers with low health literacy skills by accompanying them to provider appointments and providing health education in more readily understood terminology. Faith community nurses participate in promoting community awareness of significant health problems and building community coalitions of faith-based and service organizations to stimulate supportive public policy and interprofessional beneficial actions for improving health.

Educational Preparation for Faith Community Nursing

The faith community nurse bridges two domains and thus must be prepared in and responsible for both nursing and spiritual care. This document provides a comprehensive picture of this specialty practice as such and as part of the nursing profession. Each faith tradition may provide additional stipulations and requirements. There are designations in the specialty that indicate the level of education achieved.

Faith community nurses may also have graduate- and doctoral-level preparation in clinical nursing specialties, theology, clinical spiritual care, complementary care, palliative care, and wholistic health.

Appropriate and effective practice as an FCN requires the ability to integrate current nursing, behavioral, environmental, and spiritual knowledge with the unique spiritual beliefs and religious practices of the faith community into a program of wholistic nursing care. Such integrative practice is required regardless of the academic education of the nurse. With education, mentoring, and a collaborative practice site, an FCN may progress in levels of expertise in this specialty practice.

Faith Community Nurse

The preferred minimum preparation for a registered nurse or advanced practice registered nurse entering the specialty of faith community nursing includes:

- A baccalaureate or higher degree in nursing with academic preparation in community- or population-focused nursing

- Experience as a registered nurse using the nursing process

- Knowledge of the healthcare assets and resources of the community

- Specialized knowledge of the spiritual beliefs and practices of the faith community

- Specialized knowledge and skills to enable implementation of *Faith Community Nursing: Scope and Standards of Practice, Second Edition*

Currently, the education of all nursing students preparing for the national examination for RN licensure includes basic content on spiritual care. In addition, an increasing number of undergraduate students during their community health courses participate in clinical experiences with faith community nurses. However, because of the intentional focus on spiritual care by the faith community nurse, this educational exposure is not adequate preparation for assuming the specialty role of an FCN.

A registered nurse may prepare for the specialty of faith community nursing in several ways. Preparation may occur through accredited continuing education programs, a baccalaureate program, or graduate nursing courses.

A national Health Ministries Association (HMA) task force initiated work with the American Nurses Credentialing Center (ANCC) to begin defining criteria and a process for formal recognition of faith community nursing. Although this work is not yet completed, one of its outcomes was to establish 34 contact hours of continuing education content specific to faith community nursing as the minimum course length for the preparation for this nursing specialty.

Some educational institutions that specialize in religious education also offer relevant courses or programs of study. Collaboration between disciplines has also led to offering dual master's degrees in nursing and either theology or health ministry. Mentoring during an orientation period can also enhance faith community nursing practice. Faith communities understand, support, and often fund continuing education and spiritual development for FCNs to enhance their ability to provide spiritual care, knowing that this directly benefits a community's own programs.

Graduate-prepared or theologically prepared nurses may have certifications associated with their educational major. Currently, the motivation for a faith community nurse to pursue certification is self-directed and encouraged as part of demonstrating competence in the specialty. A specialty certification process for faith community nursing is not now available, but has been initiated as part of a pilot project. In December 2007, HMA began working with ANCC to develop a portfolio assessment process for the recognition of faith community nurses. In 2009, the portfolio assessment process was placed on hold for further study. HMA is committed to resuming work with ANCC with the intent that the portfolio process would be available for all faith community nurses interested in formal recognition by ANCC.

Advanced Practice Registered Nurse

By definition, an *advanced practice registered nurse* (APRN) is a nurse who has completed an accredited graduate-level education program preparing her or him for the role of certified nurse practitioner (CNP), certified registered nurse anesthetist (CRNA), certified nurse midwife (CNM), or clinical nurse specialist (CNS); has passed a national certification examination that measures the APRN role and population-focused competencies; maintains continued competence as evidenced by recertification; and is licensed to practice as an APRN.

An emerging role in healthcare delivery models is that of an APRN and other graduate-level prepared nurses who have acquired the additional specialized education for practice as a faith community nurse. These nurses integrate theoretical and evidence-based knowledge from graduate nursing education with the specialized education of an FCN regarding the structure, spiritual beliefs, and practices of the faith group. Examples that illustrate this role include a CNP, a wound-ostomy nurse CNS, an oncology CNS, a palliative care CNS, and a mental health CNS practicing in a faith-based community clinic.

Besides providing nursing care, these APRNs influence nursing care outcomes by serving as an advocate, consultant, or researcher in the specialty area, by providing expert consultation for spiritual leaders and other healthcare providers, and by identifying and facilitating improvements in wholistic health care.

APRN is a regulatory title and includes the four roles (CNP, CRNA, CNM, and CNS). The core competencies for education and the scope of practice are defined by the professional associations. State law and regulation further define criteria for licensure for the designated scopes of practice.

Additional Designations

National leaders of faith groups that recognize the importance of integrating this specialty nursing practice into faith communities have developed mechanisms for mentoring and providing informal and formal education in the concepts of spiritual beliefs, practices, and rituals. When such mechanisms are available within the faith group, the FCN may work with the leadership of the faith community to meet the educational and practice requirements to earn formal designation as a spiritual leader in the particular faith group.

Faith groups have different ways of designating or titling individuals who have attained an advanced level of preparation and often undergone examination to determine fitness for providing spiritual care. FCNs who achieve the requirements defined by the faith group in which they are practicing may then be given a title by the faith community indicating their achievement, such as *deacon, minister of health,* or *pastoral associate.* Titles such as these have a specialized meaning within the faith community served.

Competence and Competency in Faith Community Nursing

The American Nurses Association identifies that in the practice of nursing, "competence is definable, measurable and can be evaluated. Competence is situational, dynamic, and is both an outcome and an ongoing process. Competency is an expected level of performance that integrates knowledge, skills, abilities, and judgment in formal, informal, and reflective learning experiences. Knowledge encompasses thinking, understanding of science and humanities, professional standards of practice, and insights gained from practical experiences, personal capabilities, and leadership performance. Context determines what competencies are necessary" (ANA, 2010a, p. 12). "Formal learning most often occurs in structured, academic, and professional development environments, while informal learning can be described as experiential insights gained in work, community, home, and other settings. Reflective learning represents the recurrent thoughtful personal self-assessment, analysis, and synthesis of strengths and opportunities for improvement" (ANA, 2010a, p. 13).

Faith community nurses integrate cognitive, psychomotor, communication, interpersonal, and diagnostic skills. Their ability to act effectively involves active listening, integrity, knowledge of one's strengths and weaknesses, positive self-regard, emotional intelligence, spiritual formation, and openness to feedback. Faith community nurses must continually reassess their competencies and identify needs for additional knowledge, skills, personal growth, and integrative learning experiences.

Competence in faith community nursing practice must be evaluated by the individual nurse, peers, mentors, and faith community leaders. No single evaluation method or tool can guarantee competence. The Health Ministries Association, in its work with ANCC, has developed sources of evidence such as evidence-based case studies, spiritual journey and leadership templates, peer evaluations, faith community member narratives, and evidence of faith community nursing educational preparation and continuing education.

Settings for Practice in Faith Community Nursing

An FCN serves as a member of the interprofessional staff of a faith community, providing care to the faith community as a whole, as well as to member groups and individuals. The FCN is often the only healthcare provider responsible for practice in this nontraditional healthcare setting, although others from the faith community assist the FCN. In many circumstances, the FCN works in partnership with community agencies and healthcare systems.

Most encounters between healthcare consumers and FCNs are initiated within the faith community settings, programs, or healthcare consumers' homes. Participants in the various activities of the faith community may seek the services of the FCN. These activities include worship, education, healing prayer, special interest or support groups, programs for spiritual growth or renewal, and support services, such as shelters and soup kitchens.

A community of faith may be composed of people of all ages. The FCN provides wholistic nursing care to pediatric, adolescent, adult, and geriatric members of the faith community. The members may also represent a diverse range of physical, emotional, and cognitive development. When an individual, family, group, or the faith community as a whole experiences or desires a change in their level of physical, mental, social, environmental, or spiritual well-being, or when maintaining their current level of well-being requires nursing action, an FCN collaborates with them to develop a plan of care that incorporates communal and individual spiritual beliefs and practices.

The FCN monitors environmental, hygiene, and safety issues of faith community facilities and chooses appropriate responses in collaboration with the leadership of the faith community. Examples include hygiene and safety protocols for day care centers and nurseries; infection control during worship, health fairs, or blood drives; and protocols for response to medical emergencies. The FCN also manages physical and mental health issues, including the high levels of stress of spiritual leaders, other staff members, or faith community volunteers, with interventions that encompass spiritual support, health promotion, illness prevention, and disease management.

The needs and desires of individual members of the faith community may require that the FCN visit members in a hospital or hospice, private home, or residential facility, or accompany healthcare consumers as they use health services within the community. During these encounters the FCN may also intervene with spiritual care and provide a supportive, healing presence for both the healthcare consumer and loved ones.

The size, concerns, assets, and expectations of the faith community will guide the development of the expected role of an FCN. As a staff member, the FCN is most often supported and guided by a committee of faith community leaders and assisted by lay volunteers. With education and supervision provided by the FCN, these volunteers may assume tasks that family members would do for each other if they were available. This type of supportive team, led by the FCN, can increase safety and comfort during hospital discharge transitions and provide healthcare consumers with comprehensive support once home, helping them to recuperate more easily or to achieve peace before death.

Continued Commitment to the Profession

Because the specialty practice of faith community nursing is relatively new, each FCN needs to educate other healthcare providers and the general public about the benefits of this type of nursing care. An FCN may participate with faith community colleagues to develop collaborative efforts throughout the community by joining, for instance, a faith community nurses' group or a clergy association.

The FCN commits to lifelong learning in nursing, spiritual growth, and the beliefs and practices of the faith community. There are numerous opportunities for personal and professional growth both in and beyond the community. Major denominations support both programs and professional development. The professional organization for faith community nurses, Health Ministries Association, provides opportunities for networking and ongoing education in the practice specialty as well as with other disciplines. A variety of educational institutions and resource centers is also available around the country or online.

While the FCN may be the only healthcare provider in the faith community, the best practice cannot be provided in isolation. Personal and professional support, education opportunities, and resources are available. Accessing these will improve both the care provided to the faith community and the progress of the specialty.

Research and Faith Community Nursing

Research conducted at the National Institutes of Health and academic institutions has established a relationship between spiritual practices and health, thereby expanding the knowledge base for the specialty of faith community nursing. Findings from a variety of nonnursing disciplines provide understanding of the strong connection between spiritual well-being, participation in religious practices, and wholistic health. Involvement in a faith community provides health benefits through social support, a social identity, and a sense of power beyond one's self. Religious and spiritual practices, such as meditation, prayer, and touch, are reported to lengthen life, improve the quality of life, and improve health outcomes by enhancing psychological, physical, and spiritual well-being. Research reports may be found in the nursing literature and publications of other health professionals, as well as the professional literature focused on health ministry, chaplaincy, theology, spirituality, and spiritual care.

Research by faith community nurses to evaluate the benefits of this specialty practice is emerging. Recent studies include investigations of the measurement of clinical outcomes and the cost–benefits of faith community nursing interventions, and descriptive studies of FCN models of practice. Funding would enhance efforts to establish programs of collaborative research between practicing faith community nurses and nurse researchers that could validate and promote the wholistic health benefits of this nursing specialty in the interprofessional environment. Confirmation of positive outcomes is a major influence in funding further research and positions for faith community nurses.

Professional Trends and Issues in Faith Community Nursing

Since 1998, when faith community nursing was formally recognized by the American Nurses Association as a specialty nursing practice, there has been tremendous growth in both professional knowledge and the number of faith communities seeking such services. With this growth several issues have become more apparent.

Titling FCNs so that the title is understood across various faith traditions. This issue has been addressed with the adoption of an all-encompassing title for this specialty, *faith community nursing.* Sensitivity to the desires of individual faith communities to maintain their own internal title has also been considered. Just as each community calls their spiritual leaders by their own titles, such as rabbi, pastor, minister, or teacher, they may also call the FCN by the title they choose. However, selection of an internal title different from faith community nurse does not relieve that registered nurse from fulfilling the expectations set forth in this document.

Identifying the preparation needed for this specialty practice. This discussion is ongoing. When educational resources for this specialty were limited, nurses had minimal opportunities. With the clarification of minimum standards and an increasing awareness by nurse educators and practicing nurses of the requirements for this specialty practice, both educational expectations and opportunities have increased at all levels of nursing education. The Robert Wood Johnson Foundation and the Institute of Medicine publication, *The Future of Nursing: Leading Change, Advancing Health*, emphasizes an "action-oriented blueprint for the future of nursing" and includes recommendations for nursing educational preparation and training (2010).

Engaging other practice disciplines and faith communities in accepting this specialty nursing practice. As the number and professional activities of faith community nurses increase, so too does the recognition of these specialists by other disciplines. Faith community nurses are vital partners in advancing the nation's health initiatives, such as the Healthy People 2020 framework, to increase the quality and years of healthy life and eliminate health disparities. As members of faith communities experience the benefit of care from an FCN and share their experiences with others, the demand for these services will increase.

Developing transitional care. The recent introduction of transitional care in healthcare delivery models reflects an aspect of care that faith community nurses have been providing for members of their faith communities. Models between faith community nurses and healthcare providers are now developing in several locations as examples of collaborative community care.

Creating paid positions so that more professional nurses may choose to enter the specialty. Financial compensation for providing faith community nursing services is a complex subject familiar to those who know the history of compensation in professional nursing. In this case, the issue is complicated by three major factors:

- Lack of financial resources in many faith communities for an expansion of services

- A faith community's tradition of donating time and expertise to care for its members

- Limited objective data that demonstrate the positive health effects and benefits of faith community nursing so that external funding will be more available

As with any complex issue, addressing this situation is a multifaceted process. Some faith community nurses choose to provide care part-time or full-time, at low financial compensation if any, as part of their gift to the faith community. Others provide care so that they may demonstrate the value of this specialty practice and collect data to support the hiring of a faith community nurse for that community of faith. Some nurses, taking a broader perspective, work within faith community organizations to increase recognition of this specialty nursing practice as a form of spiritual leadership worthy of financial support. Still others encourage healthcare organizations and facilities to provide financial support to FCNs in faith communities. Given the varied dynamics of individual communities of faith, there is no one solution.

This document delineates the professional expectations associated with this specialty nursing practice. When it is considered in conjunction with *Nursing's Social Policy Statement: The Essence of the Profession* (ANA, 2010b), *Nursing: Scope and Standards of Practice, Second Edition* (ANA, 2010a), and *Code of Ethics for Nurses with Interpretive Statements* (ANA, 2001), the professional nurse receives clear guidance in the requirements for preparation and practice that best serve the public's health and the nursing profession.

Standards of Faith Community Nursing Practice

The term *faith community nurse* (FCN) is used to represent a registered nurse specializing in faith community nursing.

Standards of Practice for Faith Community Nursing

Standard 1. Assessment

The faith community nurse collects comprehensive data pertinent to the healthcare consumer's wholistic health or the situation.

COMPETENCIES

The faith community nurse:

- Collects wholistic data including but not limited to physical, functional, psychosocial, emotional, cognitive, sexual, cultural, age-related, environmental, economic, and spiritual or transpersonal assessments in a systematic and ongoing process, while honoring the uniqueness of the person and placing a particular emphasis on spiritual beliefs and practices.

- Elicits the healthcare consumer's values, preferences, expressed needs, and knowledge of the healthcare situation.

■ Involves the healthcare consumer, family, group, spiritual leader, other healthcare providers, and others, as appropriate, in wholistic data collection.

■ Identifies barriers (e.g., psychosocial, literacy, financial, cultural) to effective communication and makes appropriate adaptations.

■ Recognizes the impact of personal attitudes, values, and beliefs.

■ Assesses family dynamics and impact on healthcare consumer health and wellness.

■ Prioritizes data collection activities based on the healthcare consumer's immediate condition, or the anticipated needs of the healthcare consumer or situation.

■ Uses appropriate evidence-based assessment techniques and instruments in collecting pertinent data as a basis for wholistic care.

■ Synthesizes available data, information, and knowledge relevant to the situation to identify patterns and variances in individuals, families, groups, or the faith community as a whole.

■ Applies ethical, legal, and privacy guidelines and policies to the collection, maintenance, uses, and dissemination of data and information.

■ Recognizes healthcare consumers as the authority on their own health by honoring their care preferences.

■ Documents relevant data in a retrievable format that is both confidential and secure.

ADDITIONAL COMPETENCIES FOR THE GRADUATE-LEVEL PREPARED FAITH COMMUNITY NURSE AND THE ADVANCED PRACTICE REGISTERED NURSE

The graduate-level prepared faith community nurse or advanced practice registered nurse:

■ Initiates and interprets results from diagnostic tests relevant to the wholistic assessment of the healthcare consumer's current status.

■ Assesses the effect of interactions among individuals, family, community, and social systems on the healthcare consumer's whole (physical, mental, emotional, and spiritual) health and illness.

■ Uses evidence-based analytical models and problem-solving tools.

Standard 2. Diagnosis

The faith community nurse analyzes the assessment data to determine the diagnoses or issues.

COMPETENCIES

The faith community nurse:

- Derives the diagnoses or issues from wholistic assessment data.

- Validates the diagnoses or issues with the healthcare consumer, family, spiritual leader, and other healthcare providers, when possible and appropriate.

- Identifies actual, perceived, or potential threats and barriers to wholistic health and spiritual well-being.

- Uses standardized classification systems and clinical decision support tools, when available, in identifying diagnoses.

- Documents diagnoses in a manner that facilitates the determination of the expected outcomes and plan.

- Identifies strengths that enhance health and spiritual well-being.

ADDITIONAL COMPETENCIES FOR THE GRADUATE-LEVEL PREPARED FAITH COMMUNITY NURSE AND THE ADVANCED PRACTICE REGISTERED NURSE

The graduate-level prepared faith community nurse or advanced practice registered nurse:

- Systematically compares and contrasts clinical findings with normal and abnormal variations and developmental events in formulating a differential diagnosis.

- Utilizes complex data and information obtained during interview, wholistic assessment, examination, and diagnostic procedures in identifying diagnoses.

- Assists registered nurses in developing and maintaining competency in the diagnostic process.

Standard 3. Outcomes Identification

The faith community nurse identifies expected outcomes for a plan individualized to the healthcare consumer or the situation.

COMPETENCIES

The faith community nurse:

- Involves the healthcare consumer, family, spiritual leaders, and healthcare providers in formulating expected outcomes when possible and as appropriate.

- Derives culturally and spiritually appropriate expected outcomes from the identified diagnoses.

- Considers spiritual beliefs and practices, associated benefits, costs, risks, current scientific evidence, and clinical expertise when formulating expected outcomes.

- Defines expected outcomes in terms of the healthcare consumer and the healthcare consumer's values, spiritual and faith beliefs and practices, ethical considerations, family perspectives, cultural practices, environment, or situation with considerations such as associated benefits, risks, costs, and current scientific evidence.

- Includes a realistic time estimate for attaining expected outcomes.

- Uses collaborative discussions to develop expected outcomes that provide direction for continuity of care.

- Modifies expected outcomes based on changes in the status or desires of the healthcare consumer or on evaluation of the situation.

- Documents expected outcomes as measurable goals.

- Develops expected outcomes that facilitate attaining, maintaining, or regaining health, healing, and hope.

ADDITIONAL COMPETENCIES FOR THE GRADUATE-LEVEL PREPARED FAITH COMMUNITY NURSE AND THE ADVANCED PRACTICE REGISTERED NURSE

The graduate-level prepared faith community nurse or advanced practice registered nurse:

- Identifies expected outcomes that incorporate scientific evidence and are achievable through implementation of evidence-based practices.

- Identifies expected outcomes that incorporate cost and clinical effectiveness, healthcare consumer spiritual beliefs and satisfaction with care and quality of life, and consistency and continuity among providers.

- Differentiates outcomes that require care process interventions from those that require system-level interventions.

- Supports the use of clinical and spiritual guidelines linked to positive healthcare consumer outcomes of wholistic health and healing.

Standard 4. Planning

The faith community nurse develops a plan that prescribes strategies and alternatives to attain expected outcomes.

COMPETENCIES

The faith community nurse:

- Develops an individualized plan in partnership with the person, family, and others that considers the person's characteristics or situation, including but not limited to values, spiritual beliefs and practices, health practices, preferences, choices, developmental level, coping style, culture, religious rites, environment, and available technology.

- Establishes the plan priorities with the healthcare consumer, family, and others, as appropriate.

- Includes strategies in the plan that address each of the identified diagnoses, issues, and strengths, which may include strategies for promotion and restoration of health; spiritual enhancement; prevention of illness, injury, and disease; alleviation of suffering; and provision of supportive care for those who are dying.

- Includes strategies for health and wholeness across the life span.

- Provides for continuity within the plan.

- Incorporates an implementation pathway or timeline within the plan.

- Considers the economic impact of the plan on the healthcare consumer, family, caregivers, or other affected parties and how the faith community resources and local community resources might be of assistance.

- Integrates current scientific evidence, healthcare and wholistic health trends, and research affecting care in planning.

- Uses the plan to provide direction to other lay and professional members of the healthcare and ministry teams.

- Explores practice settings and safe space and time for the nurse and the healthcare consumer to explore suggested, potential, and alternative options.

- Defines the plan to reflect current statutes, rules, regulations, and standards.

- Modifies the plan according to the ongoing assessment of the healthcare consumer's response and other outcome indicators.

- Documents the plan in a manner that uses standardized language or recognized terminology and is understood by all participants.

- Includes strategies for wholistic health, with a focus on spirituality and growth across the life span.

ADDITIONAL COMPETENCIES FOR THE GRADUATE-LEVEL PREPARED FAITH COMMUNITY NURSE AND THE ADVANCED PRACTICE REGISTERED NURSE

The graduate-level prepared faith community nurse or advanced practice registered nurse:

- Incorporates assessment strategies, diagnostic strategies, and therapeutic interventions that reflect current evidence, including data, research, literature, and expert nursing knowledge to enhance wholistic health.

- Selects or designs nursing strategies to meet the multifaceted wholistic health needs of complex healthcare consumers.

- Includes the synthesis of healthcare consumers' values and spiritual beliefs regarding nursing and medical therapies in the plan.

- Participates in the design and development of interprofessional processes to address the situation or issue.

- Contributes to the development and continuous improvement of organizational systems that support the planning process.

- Supports the integration of clinical, human, and financial resources to enhance and complete the decision-making process.

Standard 5. Implementation

The faith community nurse implements the identified plan.

COMPETENCIES

The faith community nurse:

- Partners with the person, family, significant others, and caregiver to implement the plan in a safe, realistic, and timely manner.

- Demonstrates caring behaviors toward healthcare consumers, significant others, and groups of people receiving care.

- Utilizes technology to measure, record, and retrieve healthcare consumer data, implement the nursing process, and enhance nursing practice.

- Utilizes evidence-based interventions and treatments specific to the diagnosis or issue.

- Provides wholistic care that addresses the needs of diverse populations across the life span.

- Advocates for health care that is sensitive to the needs of healthcare consumers, with particular emphasis on the spiritual needs of diverse populations.

- Applies appropriate knowledge of major health problems and cultural diversity in implementing the plan of care.

- Applies available healthcare technologies to maximize access and optimize outcomes for healthcare consumers.

- Utilizes community and faith community resources and systems to implement the plan.

- Collaborates with healthcare providers from diverse backgrounds, spiritual leaders, caregivers, and volunteers to implement and integrate the plan.

- Accommodates different styles of communication used by healthcare consumers, families, and healthcare providers.

- Integrates traditional and complementary healthcare practices as appropriate.

- Implements the plan in a timely manner in accordance with healthcare consumer safety goals.

- Promotes the person's capacity for the optimal level of participation and problem-solving, honoring the person's choices.

- Documents implementation and any modifications, including changes or omissions, of the specified plan.

ADDITIONAL COMPETENCIES FOR THE GRADUATE-LEVEL PREPARED FAITH COMMUNITY NURSE AND THE ADVANCED PRACTICE REGISTERED NURSE

The graduate-level prepared faith community nurse or advanced practice registered nurse:

- Facilitates utilization of systems in the faith community and other community resources when necessary to implement the plan.

- Supports the development of interprofessional collaboration to implement the plan.

- Incorporates new knowledge and strategies to initiate change in faith community nursing care practices if desired outcomes are not achieved.

- Assumes responsibility for the safe and efficient implementation of the plan of care.

- Uses advanced communication skills to promote interpersonal closeness between nurses and healthcare consumers, to provide a context for open discussion of the healthcare consumer's experiences, and to improve outcomes.

- Implements the plan using principles and concepts of project or systems management.

- Fosters organizational systems that support implementation of the plan.

- Actively participates in the development and continuous improvement of systems that support the implementation of the plan.

Standard 5A. Coordination of Care

The faith community nurse coordinates care delivery.

COMPETENCIES

The faith community nurse:

- Coordinates implementation of a wholistic plan of care.

- Coordinates the health care of individuals across the life span using principles of interprofessional models of care delivery and case management.

- Organizes the components of the plan.

- Manages a healthcare consumer's care in order to maximize independence and quality of life.

- Assists the healthcare consumer to identify options for alternative care.

- Communicates with the healthcare consumer, family, and system during transitions in care.

- Advocates for the delivery of dignified and humane care by the interprofessional team.

- Documents the coordination of care.

ADDITIONAL COMPETENCIES FOR THE GRADUATE-LEVEL PREPARED FAITH COMMUNITY NURSE AND THE ADVANCED PRACTICE REGISTERED NURSE

The graduate-level prepared faith community nurse or advanced practice registered nurse:

- Provides leadership in the coordination of interprofessional health care for integrated delivery of healthcare consumer care services.

- Synthesizes data and information to prescribe necessary system and community support measures, including environmental modifications.

- Coordinates system and community resources that enhance delivery of care across continuums.

- Provides leadership in advocating for the delivery of dignified and humane care.

Standard 5B. Health Teaching and Health Promotion

The faith community nurse employs strategies to promote wholistic health, wellness, and a safe environment.

COMPETENCIES

The faith community nurse:

- Provides health teaching for individuals or groups that addresses such topics as healthy lifestyles, risk-reducing behaviors, developmental needs, activities of daily living, preventive self-care, and spiritual practices for health and healing.

- Uses health promotion and health teaching methods appropriate to the situation and the healthcare consumer's values, beliefs, health practices, developmental level, learning needs, readiness and ability to learn, language preference, spirituality, culture, and socioeconomic status.

- Seeks ongoing opportunities for feedback and evaluation of the effectiveness of the strategies used.

- Uses information technologies to communicate health promotion and disease prevention information to the healthcare consumer in a variety of settings.

- Provides healthcare consumers with information about intended effects and potential adverse effects of proposed therapies.

- Teaches activities that strengthen the body–mind–spirit connection, such as meditation, prayer, and guided imagery.

- Evaluates health information resources for use in faith community nursing for accuracy, readability, and comprehensibility by healthcare consumers, and compatibility with the healthcare consumers' spiritual beliefs and practices.

ADDITIONAL COMPETENCIES FOR THE GRADUATE-LEVEL PREPARED FAITH COMMUNITY NURSE AND THE ADVANCED PRACTICE REGISTERED NURSE

The graduate-level prepared faith community nurse or advanced practice registered nurse:

- Synthesizes empirical evidence on spiritual practices, risk behaviors, learning theories, behavioral change theories, motivational theories, epidemiology, and other related theories and frameworks when designing wholistic health information and healthcare consumer education.

- Conducts personalized health teaching and counseling considering comparative effectiveness research recommendations.

- Designs health information and healthcare consumer education appropriate to the healthcare consumer's spiritual beliefs and practices, cultural values and beliefs, developmental level, learning needs, readiness to learn, and readiness to experience new spiritual practices.

- Evaluates health information resources, such as the Internet, for accuracy, readability, and comprehensibility to help healthcare consumers to access quality health information that is compatible with their spiritual beliefs and practices.

- Engages faith-based organizations, consumer alliances, and advocacy groups, as appropriate, in health teaching and health promotion activities that are restorative, supportive, and promotive in nature.

- Provides anticipatory guidance to individuals, families, and groups in the faith communities to promote health and prevent or reduce the risk of health problems.

Standard 5C. Consultation

The faith community nurse provides consultation to facilitate understanding and influence the specified plan of care, enhance the abilities of others, and effect change.

COMPETENCIES

The faith community nurse:

- Initiates consultation with chaplains and spiritual leaders for resources, guidance, and support within the spiritual realm.

- Facilitates the effectiveness of a consultation by involving the healthcare consumer in decision-making and role negotiation.

- Consults with APRNs and other healthcare providers.

- Communicates consultation recommendations.

ADDITIONAL COMPETENCIES FOR THE GRADUATE-LEVEL PREPARED FAITH COMMUNITY NURSE AND THE ADVANCED PRACTICE REGISTERED NURSE

The graduate-level prepared faith community nurse or advanced practice registered nurse:

- Synthesizes spiritual practices, organizational structure, and beliefs of the faith group; clinical data; theoretical frameworks; and evidence when providing consultation.

- Facilitates the effectiveness of a consultation by involving the healthcare consumer or their designee in decision-making and negotiating role responsibilities for each member of the faith community.

- Communicates consultation recommendations effectively to influence the identified plan, facilitate understanding, enhance the work of the faith community team, and effect lasting change.

- Provides, structures, and maintains a safe therapeutic environment in collaboration with healthcare consumers, families, and other healthcare clinicians.

Standard 5D. Prescriptive Authority and Treatment

The advanced practice registered nurse uses prescriptive authority, procedures, referrals, treatments, and therapies in accordance with state and federal laws and regulations.

COMPETENCIES FOR THE ADVANCED PRACTICE REGISTERED NURSE

The advanced practice registered nurse:

- Prescribes evidence-based treatments, therapies, and procedures considering the healthcare consumer's comprehensive healthcare needs and spiritual needs, beliefs, and practices.

- Prescribes therapies, including those that strengthen the body–mind–spirit connection such as meditation, prayer, guided imagery, and various rituals of worship.

- Prescribes pharmacological agents according to a current knowledge of pharmacology and physiology.

- Prescribes specific pharmacological agents or treatments based on clinical indicators, the healthcare consumer's status and needs, and the results of diagnostic and laboratory tests.

- Evaluates therapeutic and potential adverse effects of pharmacological and nonpharmacological treatments.

- Provides healthcare consumers with information about intended effects and potential adverse effects of proposed prescriptive therapies.

- Provides information about costs and alternative treatments and procedures, as appropriate.

- Evaluates and incorporates complementary and alternative therapy into education and practice.

Standard 6. Evaluation

The faith community nurse evaluates progress toward attainment of outcomes.

COMPETENCIES

The faith community nurse:

- Conducts a wholistic, systematic, ongoing, and criterion-based evaluation of the outcomes in relation to the structures and processes prescribed by the plan and the indicated timeline.

- Collaborates with the healthcare consumer and others involved in the care or situation in the evaluative process.

- Evaluates, in partnership with the healthcare consumer, the effectiveness of the planned strategies in relation to the healthcare consumer's responses and attainment of expected outcomes.

- Uses ongoing assessment data to revise the diagnoses, the outcomes, the plan, and the plan's implementation as needed.

- Disseminates the results to the healthcare consumer and others involved in the care or situation, as appropriate, in accordance with state and federal laws and regulations.

- Participates in assessing and ensuring the responsible and appropriate use of interventions in order to minimize unwarranted or unwanted treatment and healthcare consumer suffering.

- Documents the results of the evaluation, including results from the faith or spiritual realm.

ADDITIONAL COMPETENCIES FOR THE GRADUATE-LEVEL PREPARED FAITH COMMUNITY NURSE AND THE ADVANCED PRACTICE REGISTERED NURSE

The graduate-level prepared faith community nurse or the advanced practice registered nurse:

- Evaluates the accuracy of the diagnosis and effectiveness of the interventions in relation to the healthcare consumer's attainment of expected outcomes.

■ Uses spiritual assessment tools to identify the influence of the healthcare consumer's and family's views of health and healing on attainment of outcomes.

■ Synthesizes the results of the evaluation analyses to determine the impact of the plan on the affected healthcare consumers, families, groups, faith communities and institutions, collegial networks, organizations, and geopolitical communities.

■ Adapts the plan of care as well as policy and procedures of practice for the trajectory of treatment, when appropriate, based on evaluation of response by individuals and groups in faith communities.

■ Uses the results of the evaluation to make or recommend process or structural changes, including policy, procedure, or protocol revision, as appropriate.

■ Uses the results of the evaluation analyses to increase awareness beyond the individual faith community of the wholistic health benefits and spiritual care provided through faith community nursing.

Standards of Professional Performance for Faith Community Nursing

Standard 7. Ethics

The faith community nurse practices ethically.

COMPETENCIES

The faith community nurse:

- Uses *Code of Ethics for Nurses with Interpretive Statements* (ANA, 2001) to guide practice.

- Delivers care in a manner that preserves and protects the healthcare consumer's autonomy, dignity, rights, and spiritual beliefs and practices.

- Recognizes the centrality of the healthcare consumer and family as core members of any healthcare team.

- Upholds healthcare consumer confidentiality within religious, legal, and regulatory parameters.

- Assists healthcare consumers in self-determination and informed decision-making.

- Maintains a therapeutic and professional healthcare consumer–nurse relationship within appropriate professional role boundaries.

- Contributes to resolving ethical issues of healthcare consumers, colleagues, community groups, or systems, and other stakeholders.

- Takes appropriate action regarding instances of illegal, unethical, or inappropriate behavior that can endanger or jeopardize the best interests of the healthcare consumer or situation.

- Speaks up as appropriate to question healthcare practice when necessary for safety and quality improvement.

- Advocates for equitable healthcare consumer care.

- Empowers healthcare consumers in developing skills for self-advocacy in support of their spiritual beliefs and practices.

- Incorporates ethical and moral theories, principles, and models in processes of care planning and delivery.

- Acknowledges and respects tenets of the faith and spiritual belief system of a healthcare consumer.

ADDITIONAL COMPETENCIES FOR THE GRADUATE-LEVEL PREPARED FAITH COMMUNITY NURSE AND THE ADVANCED PRACTICE REGISTERED NURSE

The graduate-level prepared faith community nurse or the advanced practice registered nurse:

- Provides information on the risks, benefits, and outcomes of healthcare regimens to allow informed decision-making by the healthcare consumer, including informed consent and informed refusal.

- Participates in interprofessional teams that address ethical risks, benefits, and outcomes of programs and decisions that affect health and healthcare delivery.

- Mentors interprofessional teams in processes of ethical decision-making.

- Advocates for equitable healthcare consumer care.

Standard 8. Education

The faith community nurse attains knowledge and competence that reflect current nursing practice.

COMPETENCIES

The faith community nurse:

- Participates in ongoing educational activities related to appropriate knowledge bases, professional issues, and spiritual care.

- Demonstrates a commitment to lifelong learning through self-reflection and inquiry to address learning and personal growth needs.

- Seeks experiences that reflect current practice to maintain knowledge, skills, abilities, and judgment in clinical practice or role performance for faith community nursing.

- Acquires knowledge and skills appropriate to the role, population, specialty of faith community nursing, setting, or situation.

- Seeks formal and independent learning experience to develop and maintain clinical, professional, and theological skills and knowledge.

- Identifies learning needs based on nursing knowledge, the various roles the nurse may assume, and the changing needs of the population.

- Participates in formal or informal consultations to address issues in nursing practice as an application of education and knowledge base.

- Shares educational findings, experiences, and ideas with peers.

- Contributes to a work environment conducive to the education of healthcare professionals.

- Maintains professional records that provide evidence of competence and lifelong learning.

ADDITIONAL COMPETENCIES FOR THE GRADUATE-LEVEL PREPARED FAITH COMMUNITY NURSE AND THE ADVANCED PRACTICE REGISTERED NURSE

The graduate-level prepared faith community nurse or the advanced practice registered nurse:

- Uses current healthcare research findings and other evidence to expand clinical and professional knowledge in order to better combine the two domains, nursing and spiritual care, into one practice role.

Standard 9. Evidence-Based Practice and Research

The faith community nurse integrates evidence and research findings into practice.

COMPETENCIES

The faith community nurse:

- Utilizes current evidence-based nursing knowledge, including research findings, to guide practice.

- Incorporates evidence when initiating changes in nursing practice.

- Participates, as appropriate to education level and position, in the formulation of evidence-based practice through research.

- Shares personal or third-party research findings with colleagues and peers.

ADDITIONAL COMPETENCIES FOR THE GRADUATE-LEVEL PREPARED FAITH COMMUNITY NURSE AND THE ADVANCED PRACTICE REGISTERED NURSE

The graduate-level prepared faith community nurse or the advanced practice registered nurse:

- Contributes to nursing knowledge by conducting or synthesizing research that discovers, examines, and evaluates knowledge, theories, criteria, and creative approaches to integrating spiritual care and nursing care in a faith community.

- Disseminates research findings through interdisciplinary activities such as presentations, publications, consultations, and journal clubs.

- Cultivates a climate of research and clinical inquiry.

Standard 10. Quality of Practice

The faith community nurse contributes to quality nursing practice.

COMPETENCIES

The faith community nurse:

- Demonstrates quality by documenting the application of the nursing process in a responsible, accountable, and ethical manner.

- Uses creativity, innovation in faith community nursing practice, and the resources of clergy, chaplains, hospice staff, and other colleagues to improve care delivery.

- Participates in quality improvement activities for faith community nursing. Such activities may include:

  - Identifying aspects of practice important for quality monitoring.

  - Using indicators to monitor quality and effectiveness of faith community nursing practice.

  - Collecting data to monitor quality and effectiveness of faith community nursing practice.

  - Analyzing quality data to identify opportunities for improving faith community nursing practice.

  - Formulating recommendations to improve faith community nursing practice or outcomes.

  - Implementing activities to enhance the quality of faith community nursing practice.

  - Developing, implementing, and evaluating policies, procedures, and guidelines to improve the quality of care.

  - Participating on and leading interprofessional teams to evaluate clinical care or health services.

  - Participating in and leading efforts to minimize costs and unnecessary duplication.

- Identifying problems that occur in day-to-day work routines in order to correct process inefficiencies.

- Analyzing factors related to quality, safety, and effectiveness.

- Analyzing organizational systems in the faith community for barriers to quality healthcare consumer outcomes.

- Implementing processes to remove or weaken barriers within the organizational systems in healthcare settings and the faith community.

- Participating in prayer, spiritual direction, and other intentional spiritual practices to enhance sustainability, personal growth, and skills as a spiritual care provider.

ADDITIONAL COMPETENCIES FOR THE GRADUATE-LEVEL PREPARED FAITH COMMUNITY NURSE AND THE ADVANCED PRACTICE REGISTERED NURSE

The graduate-level prepared faith community nurse or the advanced practice registered nurse:

- Provides leadership in the design and implementation of quality improvement activities.

- Designs innovations to effect change in practice and improve health outcomes.

- Evaluates the practice environment and quality of nursing care rendered in relation to existing evidence, identifying opportunities for the generation and use of research.

- Develops indicators to monitor quality and effectiveness of faith community nursing practice.

Standard 11. Communication

The faith community nurse communicates effectively in a variety of formats in all areas of practice.

COMPETENCIES

The faith community nurse:

- Assesses communication format preferences of healthcare consumers, families, and colleagues.

- Assesses his or her own communication skills in encounters with healthcare consumers, families, and colleagues.

- Seeks continuous improvement of his or her own communication and conflict-resolution skills.

- Conveys information to healthcare consumers, families, the interprofessional team, and others in communication formats that promote accuracy.

- Questions the rationale supporting routine approaches to care processes and decisions when they do not appear to be in the best interest of the healthcare consumer.

- Discloses observations or concerns related to hazards and errors in care or the practice environment to the appropriate level.

- Maintains communication with other providers to minimize risks associated with transfers and transition in care delivery.

- Contributes her or his own professional perspective in discussions with the interprofessional team.

Standard 12. Leadership

The faith community nurse demonstrates leadership in the professional practice setting and the profession.

COMPETENCIES

The faith community nurse:

- Oversees the nursing care given by others while retaining accountability for the quality of care given to the healthcare consumer.

- Abides by the vision, associated goals, and plan to implement and measure progress of an individual healthcare consumer or progress within the context of the healthcare organization.

- Demonstrates a commitment to continuous, lifelong learning, education, and spiritual growth for self and others.

- Mentors colleagues in relation to spirituality for the advancement of nursing practice, the profession, and quality health care.

- Treats colleagues with respect, trust, and dignity.

- Develops communication and conflict resolution skills.

- Participates in professional organizations.

- Communicates effectively with the healthcare consumer and colleagues.

- Seeks ways to advance nursing autonomy and accountability.

- Participates in efforts to influence healthcare policy involving healthcare consumers and the profession.

- Serves in key leadership roles in the faith community by participating on committees, councils, and health ministry administrative teams.

ADDITIONAL COMPETENCIES FOR THE GRADUATE-LEVEL PREPARED FAITH COMMUNITY NURSE AND THE ADVANCED PRACTICE REGISTERED NURSE

The graduate-level prepared faith community nurse or the advanced practice registered nurse:

- Influences decision-making bodies to improve the professional practice environment and healthcare consumer outcomes.

- Provides direction to enhance the effectiveness of the interprofessional team.

- Promotes advanced practice nursing and role development by interpreting its role for healthcare consumers, families, and others.

- Models expert practice to interprofessional team members and healthcare consumers.

- Mentors colleagues in the acquisition of clinical knowledge, skills, abilities, ethics, and judgment.

- Leads in enhancing the effectiveness of the interprofessional team.

- Promotes advancement of the profession through activities such as publishing, public speaking, and participation in professional organizations.

- Initiates revision of protocols or guidelines for community care to reflect evidence-based faith community nursing practice, to reflect the benefit of care management by faith community nurses, or to address emerging problems.

- Analyzes the economic, legal, regulatory, and political factors that influence healthcare delivery.

- Designs innovations to effect change in faith community nursing practice and improve the outcomes of wholistic health and healing.

Standard 13. Collaboration

The faith community nurse collaborates with the healthcare consumer, family, and others in the conduct of nursing practice.

COMPETENCIES

The faith community nurse:

- Partners with others to effect change and produce positive outcomes through the sharing of knowledge about the healthcare consumer and the situation.

- Communicates with the healthcare consumer, family, groups, spiritual leaders, hospital and hospice chaplains, and other healthcare providers regarding healthcare consumer care and the faith community nurse's role in the provision of that care.

- Promotes conflict management and engagement.

- Participates in consensus building or conflict resolution in the context of healthcare consumer care within faith community and healthcare settings.

- Applies group process and negotiation techniques with healthcare consumers and colleagues.

- Adheres to standards and applicable codes of conduct that govern behavior among peers and colleagues to create a work environment that promotes cooperation, respect, and trust.

- Cooperates in creating a documented plan focused on outcomes and decisions related to care and delivery of services that indicates communication with healthcare consumers, families, and others.

- Engages in teamwork and team-building processes.

- Documents referrals, including hospice and other provisions for continuity of care outside the faith community.

ADDITIONAL COMPETENCIES FOR THE GRADUATE-LEVEL PREPARED FAITH COMMUNITY NURSE AND THE ADVANCED PRACTICE REGISTERED NURSE

The graduate-level prepared faith community nurse or the advanced practice registered nurse:

- Partners with other disciplines to enhance healthcare consumer outcomes through interprofessional activities, such as education, consultation, management, technological development, or research opportunities.

- Invites the contribution of the healthcare consumer, family, and team members in order to achieve optimal outcomes.

- Leads in establishing, improving, and sustaining collaborative relationships to achieve safe, quality healthcare consumer care.

- Documents plan-of-care communications, rationales for plan-of-care changes, and collaborative discussions to improve healthcare consumer outcomes.

- Participates on interprofessional teams that contribute to role development and, directly or indirectly, advance nursing practice and health services.

Standard 14. Professional Practice Evaluation

The faith community nurse evaluates his or her own nursing practice in relation to professional practice standards and guidelines, relevant statutes, rules, and regulations.

COMPETENCIES

The faith community nurse's practice reflects the application of knowledge of current practice standards, guidelines, statutes, rules, and regulations.

The faith community nurse:

- Provides age-appropriate and developmentally appropriate care in a spiritually, culturally, and ethnically sensitive manner.

- Engages in self-evaluation of practice regularly, identifying areas of strength as well as areas in which professional development would be beneficial.

- Obtains informal feedback regarding her or his own spiritual care and nursing practice from healthcare consumers, peers, spiritual leaders, health committee members, faith community volunteers, professional colleagues, and others.

- Participates in systematic formal review, as appropriate.

- Takes action to achieve goals identified during the evaluation process.

- Provides evidence for practice decisions and actions as part of the informal and formal evaluation processes.

- Interacts with peers and colleagues to enhance her or his own professional nursing practice or role performance.

- Provides peers with formal or informal constructive feedback regarding their practice or role performance.

ADDITIONAL COMPETENCIES FOR THE GRADUATE-LEVEL PREPARED FAITH COMMUNITY NURSE AND THE ADVANCED PRACTICE REGISTERED NURSE

The graduate-level prepared faith community nurse or the advanced practice registered nurse:

- Engages in a formal process seeking feedback regarding her or his own practice from healthcare consumers, peers, professional colleagues, and others.

Standard 15. Resource Utilization

The faith community nurse utilizes appropriate resources to plan and provide nursing services that are safe, effective, and financially responsible.

COMPETENCIES

The faith community nurse:

- Assesses individual healthcare consumer care needs and resources available to achieve desired outcomes.

- Identifies healthcare consumer care needs, potential for harm, complexity of the task, and desired outcome when considering resource allocation.

- Delegates elements of care to appropriate healthcare workers in accordance with any applicable legal or policy parameters or principles.

- Identifies the evidence when evaluating resources.

- Advocates for resources, including technology, that enhance nursing practice.

- Modifies practice when necessary to promote a positive interface between healthcare consumers, care providers, and technology.

- Assists the healthcare consumer and family in identifying and securing appropriate and available resources to address health and spiritually related needs across the healthcare continuum.

- Assists the healthcare consumer and family in factoring costs, risks, and benefits in decisions about treatment and care.

- Develops innovative solutions and applies strategies to obtain appropriate resources for faith community nursing care.

ADDITIONAL COMPETENCIES FOR THE GRADUATE-LEVEL PREPARED FAITH COMMUNITY NURSE AND THE ADVANCED PRACTICE REGISTERED NURSE

The graduate-level prepared faith community nurse or the advanced practice registered nurse:

- Utilizes organizational and community resources to formulate interprofessional plans of care.

- Formulates innovative solutions for healthcare consumer care problems that utilize resources effectively and maintain quality.

- Designs evaluation strategies that demonstrate cost-effectiveness, cost–benefit, and efficiency factors associated with nursing practice.

Standard 16. Environmental Health

The faith community nurse practices in an environmentally safe and healthy manner.

COMPETENCIES

The faith community nurse:

- Attains knowledge of environmental health concepts, such as implementation of environmental health strategies.

- Promotes a practice environment that reduces environmental health risks for workers and healthcare consumers.

- Assesses the practice environment for such factors as sound, odor, noise, and light that threaten health.

- Advocates for the judicious and appropriate use of products in health care.

- Communicates environmental health risks and exposure reduction strategies to healthcare consumers, families, colleagues, faith communities, and broader communities.

- Utilizes scientific evidence to determine if a product or treatment is an environmental threat.

- Participates in strategies to promote healthy communities.

- Addresses environmental health risks in the home, workplace, faith community, and healthcare setting.

- Advocates for environmental health and social justice, including a commitment to the health of vulnerable populations.

ADDITIONAL COMPETENCIES FOR THE GRADUATE-LEVEL PREPARED FAITH COMMUNITY NURSE AND THE ADVANCED PRACTICE REGISTERED NURSE

The graduate-level prepared faith community nurse or the advanced practice registered nurse:

- Creates partnerships that promote sustainable environmental health policies and conditions.

- Analyzes the impact of social, political, and economic influences on the environment and human health exposures.

- Critically evaluates the manner in which environmental health issues are presented by the popular media.

- Advocates for implementation of environmental principles for nursing practice.

- Identifies patterns of comorbidities among family and community members suggesting environmental etiologies.

Glossary

Assessment. A systematic, dynamic process by which a faith community registered nurse, through interaction with the healthcare consumer, family, groups, communities, populations, spiritual leaders, and healthcare providers, collects and analyzes data. In addition to spiritual dimensions, asssessment by the faith community registered nurse may include the following dimensions: physical, psychological, sociocultural, cognitive, functional abilities, developmental, economic, environmental, and lifestyle.

Caregiver. A person who provides direct care for another, such as a child, a dependent adult, or a person with a disability, chronic illness, or spiritual distress.

Code of ethics. A succinct list of provisions that makes explicit the primary goals, values, and obligations of the profession.

Competency. An expected and measurable level of nursing performance that integrates knowledge, skills, abilities, and judgment and that is based on established scientific knowledge and expectations for nursing practice.

Continuity of care. An interdisciplinary process that includes healthcare consumers, families, significant others, and appropriate members of a faith community in the development of a coordinated plan of care. This process facilitates the healthcare consumer's transition between settings and healthcare providers, based on changing needs and available resources.

Diagnosis. A clinical judgment about the healthcare consumer's response to actual, perceived, or potential health concerns or needs. The diagnosis provides the basis for determining a plan to achieve desired outcomes, to establish priorities, and to develop a plan of action with the healthcare consumer. Faith community registered nurses utilize nursing diagnoses or medical diagnoses depending on their education, clinical preparation, and legal authority.

Disease. A biological or psychosocial disorder of structure or function in a healthcare consumer, especially a disorder that produces specific signs or symptoms or that affects a specific part of the body, mind, or spirit.

Documentation. The recording of the assessment, plan of care, interventions, and evaluation of outcomes in a retrievable format that is confidential and secure for the healthcare consumer to facilitate continuity in meeting desired health outcomes.

Environment. The atmosphere, milieu, or conditions in which an individual lives, works, plays, or carries out his or her faith practices.

Evaluation. The process of determining the progress toward attainment of expected outcomes and the satisfaction of the healthcare consumer with those outcomes for the purpose of modifying the plan. Outcomes include the effectiveness of care, when addressing one's own practice.

Evidence-based practice. A process founded on the collection, interpretation, and integration of valid, important, and applicable healthcare consumer reported, clinician-observed, and research-derived evidence. The best available evidence, moderated by healthcare consumer circumstances and preferences, is applied to improve the quality of clinical judgments.

Faith community. An organization of groups, families, and individuals who share common values, beliefs, religious doctrine, and faith practices that influence their lives, generally in the setting of a church, synagogue, temple, mosque or faith-based agency, and that functions as a healthcare consumer system, providing a setting for faith community nursing.

Faith community nurse (FCN). A registered professional nurse who is actively licensed in a given state and who serves as a member of the staff of a faith community. The FCN promotes health as wholeness of the faith community, its groups, families, and individual members through the practice of nursing as defined by that state's nurse practice act in the jurisdiction in which the FCN practices and the standards of practice set forth in this document.

Faith community nursing. The specialized practice of professional nursing that focuses on the intentional care of the spirit as well as on the promotion of wholistic health and prevention or minimization of illness within the context of a faith community.

Faith group. A specific denomination or sect within a faith tradition.

Family. Family of origin or significant others as identified by a healthcare consumer, who may refer to some or all of the members of a faith community as part of their family.

Group. A number of people sharing something in common, such as an interest, activity, or spiritual beliefs and practices.

Healing. The process of integrating the body, mind, and spirit to bring about wholeness, health, and a sense of spiritual well-being, although the healthcare consumer's disease may not be cured.

Health. The experience of wholeness, salvation, or shalom. The integration of the spiritual, physical, psychological, emotional, and social aspects of the healthcare consumer to create a sense of harmony with self, others, the environment, and a higher power. Health may be experienced in the presence or absence of disease or injury.

Healthcare consumer. The person, client, family, group, community, or population who is the focus of attention and to whom the registered nurse is providing services as sanctioned by the state regulatory bodies. The term *healthcare consumer* is used to provide consistency and brevity, bearing in mind that other terms, such as *client, individual, family, groups, community,* or *population,* might be better choices in some instances.

- When the healthcare consumer is an individual, the focus is on the health state, problems, or needs of the individual.

- When the healthcare consumer is a family or group, the focus is on the health of the unit as a whole or the reciprocal effects of the individual's health on the other members of the unit.

- When the healthcare consumer is a community or population, the focus is on personal and environmental health and the health risks of the community or population.

Healthcare providers. Individuals with special expertise who provide healthcare services or assistance to healthcare consumers. They may include nurses, physicians, spiritual leaders, psychologists, social workers, nutritionists/dietitians, and various therapists.

Health ministry. The promotion of health and healing as part of the mission and service of a faith community to its members and the community it serves.

Health promotion. Activities and interventions that healthcare consumers undertake to achieve desired health outcomes. Health promotion outcomes may be primary (the prevention of disease and injury); secondary (the early detection and appropriate intervention in illness or brokenness); or tertiary (the promotion of wholeness and sense of well-being when curing may not occur).

Illness. The subjective experience of discomfort, brokenness; the disintegration of body, mind, spirit; disharmony with others, the environment, or a higher power.

Implementation. Activities such as teaching, monitoring, providing, praying, leading meditation, counseling, delegating, and coordinating. Carrying out of a plan of action in a spiritual, caring relationship that provides the information, skills, motivation, spiritual or faith tradition rituals, and resources necessary to empower the healthcare consumer to achieve desired health outcomes.

Interprofessional. Reliant on overlapping knowledge, skills, and abilities of each team member and discipline, resulting in synergistic effects where outcomes are enhanced and more comprehensive than the simple aggregation of any team member's individual efforts.

Patient. See *Healthcare consumer.*

Peer review/evaluation. A collegial, systematic, and periodic process by which faith community nurses are held accountable for their practice and that fosters the refinement of one's knowledge, skills, and decision-making.

Plan. A comprehensive outline of the components that need to be completed to attain mutually identified and expected healthcare consumer outcomes.

Quality of care. The degree to which health services for healthcare consumers, families, groups, communities, or populations increase the likelihood of desired outcomes and are consistent with current professional knowledge.

Registered nurse (RN). An individual registered or licensed by a state, commonwealth, territory, government, or other regulatory body to practice as a registered nurse.

Restorative practices. Nursing interventions that mitigate the impact of illness or disease.

Scope of nursing practice. The description of the *who, what, where, when, why,* and *how* of nursing practice that addresses the range of nursing practice activities common to all registered nurses. When considered in conjunction with the Standards of Professional Nursing Practice and the Code of Ethics for Nurses, comprehensively describes the competent level of nursing common to all registered nurses.

Self-care. Actions a faith community, group, family, or individual take to attain desired wholistic health outcomes when they possess the requisite knowledge, skills, ability, resources, motivation, encouragement, and support.

Spiritual care. The practical expression of presence, guidance, and interventions, individual or communal, to support, nurture, or encourage an individual's or group's ability to achieve wholeness; health; personal, spiritual, and social well-being; integration of body, mind, and spirit; and a sense of connection to self, others, and a higher power.

Spiritual leader. An individual recognized and authorized by a faith community, such as a clergyperson (pastor, priest, rabbi, shaman), chaplain, or lay minister, who guides and inspires others in the study and nurture of their spiritual beliefs and application of spiritual practices.

Standard. An authoritative statement defined and promoted by the profession by which the quality of practice, service, or education can be evaluated.

Supportive practices. Nursing interventions that are oriented toward modification of relationships or the environment to support health.

Transitional care. Actions of faith community nurses and other healthcare providers designed to ensure the coordination and continuity of health care for healthcare consumers during movement between hospitals, sub-acute and post-acute nursing facilities, the healthcare consumer's home, primary and specialty care offices, and long-term care facilities as their condition and care needs change during the course of a chronic or acute illness.

Well-being. An individual's perception of her or his own wholistic health.

Wholistic. Based on an understanding that a healthcare consumer is an interconnected unity and that physical, mental, social, environmental, and spiritual factors need to be included in any interventions. The whole system, whether referring to a human being or a faith community, is greater than the sum of its parts. The preferred term when referring to the type of care provided by a faith community nurse.

References and Bibliography

American Nurses Association. (2001). *Code of ethics for nurses with interpretive statements*. Washington, DC: Nursesbooks.org.

American Nurses Association. (2010a). *Nursing: Scope and standards of practice, second edition*. Silver Spring, MD: Nursesbooks.org.

American Nurses Association. (2010b). *Nursing's social policy statement: The essence of the profession*. Silver Spring, MD: Nursesbooks.org.

Brown, A. R., Coppola, P., Giacona, M., Petriches, A., & Stockwell, M. A. (2009). Faith community nursing demonstrates good stewardship of community benefit dollars through cost savings and cost avoidance. *Family and Community Health, 32*(4), 330–338. doi.10.1097/FCH.0b013e3181b91f93

Catanzaro, A. M., Meador, K. G., Koenig, H. G., Kuchibhatla, M., & Clipp, E. C. (2007). Congregational health ministries: A national study of pastors' views. *Public Health Nursing, 24*(1), 6–17. doi:10.1111/j.1525-1446.2006.00602.x

Chase-Ziolek, M. (2005). *Health, healing, and wholeness: Engaging congregations in ministries of health*. Cleveland, OH: Pilgrim Press.

Chase-Ziolek, M., & Iris, M. (2002). Nurses' perspectives on the distinctive aspects of providing nursing care in a congregational setting. *Journal of Community Health Nursing, 19*(3), 173–186.

Coleman, E. A., & Boult, C. E. (2003). Improving the quality of transitional care for persons with complex care needs. *Journal of the American Geriatrics Society, 51*(4), 556–557.

Donahue, M. P. (1996). *Nursing, the finest art: An illustrated history* (2nd ed.). St. Louis, MO: Mosby.

Dunn, H. L. (1959). High-level wellness for man and society. *Journal of Public Health, 49*(6), 786–792.

Dyess, S., Chase, S. K, & Newlin, K. (2010). State of research for faith community nursing 2009. *Journal of Religion and Health, 49*(2), 188–199.

Health Ministries Association and American Nurses Association. (1998). *Scope and standards of parish nursing practice*. Washington, DC: American Nurses Publishing.

Hickman, J. S. (2006). *Faith community nursing*. Philadelphia: Lippincott, Williams and Wilkins.

Institute of Medicine. (2010). *The future of nursing: Leading change, advancing health*. Washington, DC: National Academy of Sciences.

Koenig, H. G., McCullough, M. E., & Larson, D. B. (2001). *The handbook of religion and health*. Oxford, England: Oxford University Press.

Levin, J. (2002). *God, faith, and health: Exploring the spirituality-healing connection*. New York, NY: John Wiley and Sons.

Mayernik, D., Resick, L. K., Skomo, M. L., & Mandock, K. (2010). Parish nurse-initiated interdisciplinary mobile health care delivery project. *Journal of Obstetric, Gynecologic, and Neonatal Nursing, 39*(2), 227–234.

North American Nursing Diagnosis Association (NANDA). (2009). *Nursing diagnoses: Definitions and classification 2008–2009*. Philadelphia: NANDA International.

Puchalski, C. M., & Ferrell, B. (2010). *Making health care whole: Integrating spirituality into patient care*. West Conshohocken, PA: Templeton Press.

Rethemeyer, A., & Wehling, B. A. (2004). How are we doing? Measuring the effectiveness of parish nursing. *Journal of Christian Nursing, 21*(2), 10–12.

Smucker, C. J., & Weinberg, L. (2009). *Faith community nursing: Developing a quality practice.* Silver Spring, MD: Nursesbooks.org.

Solari-Twadell, P. A., & Hackbarth, D. P. (2010). Evidence for a new paradigm of the ministry of parish nursing practice using the nursing intervention classification system. *Nursing Outlook, 58*(2), 69–75.

Weis, D., Schank, M., Coenen, A., & Matheus, R. (2002). Parish nurse practice with client aggregates. *Journal of Community Health Nursing, 19*(2), 105–113.

Appendix A.

Faith Community Nursing:
Scope and Standards
of Practice (2005)

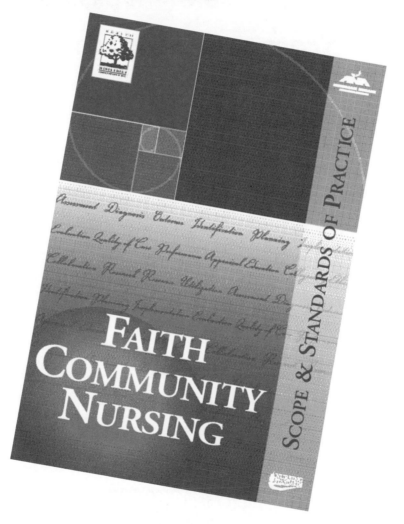

This appendix is not current and is of historical significance only.

This appendix is not current and is of historical significance only.

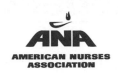

FAITH COMMUNITY NURSING:

SCOPE AND STANDARDS

OF PRACTICE

AMERICAN NURSES ASSOCIATION

SILVER SPRING, MD

2005

This appendix is not current and is of historical significance only.

Library of Congress Cataloging-in-Publication data

Health Ministries Association.
 Faith community nursing : scope and standards of practice / Health Ministries Association.
  p. ; cm.
 Includes bibliographical references and index.
 ISBN-13: 978-1-55810-228-6
 ISBN-10: 1-55810-228-0
 1. Parish nursing—Standards—United States. 2. Community health nursing—Standards—United States. I. American Nurses Association. II. Title.
 [DNLM: 1. Community Health Nursing—standards. 2. Spirituality. 3. Cultural Diversity. 4. Nursing Process—standards. 5. Religion. WY 87 H434f 2005]
 RT120.P37H43 2005
 610.73'43—dc22   2005015923

The American Nurses Association (ANA) is a national professional association. This ANA publication—*Faith Community Nursing: Scope and Standards of Practice*—reflects the thinking of the nursing profession on various issues and should be reviewed in conjunction with state board of nursing policies and practices. State law, rules, and regulations govern the practice of nursing, while *Faith Community Nursing: Scope and Standards of Practice* guides nurses in the application of their professional skills and responsibilities.

Health Ministries Association (HMA), a non-profit organization, is a support network for people of faith who promote whole-person health through faith groups in the communities they serve. By providing information, guidelines, and resources, HMA assists and encourages individuals, called health ministers, as they develop whole-person health programs, utilize community resources, and educate others on the interdependent health of body, mind and spirit.

Published by nursesbooks.org
The Publishing Program of ANA

American Nurses Association
8515 Georgia Avenue, Suite 400
Silver Spring, MD 20910-3492
1-800-274-4ANA
http://www.nursesbooks.org/

ANA is the only full-service professional organization representing the nation's 2.7 million Registered Nurses through its 54 constituent member associations. ANA advances the nursing profession by fostering high standards of nursing practice, promoting the economic and general welfare of nurses in the workplace, projecting a positive and realistic view of nursing, and lobbying the Congress and regulatory agencies on healthcare issues affecting nurses and the public.

ISBN 978-1-55810-228-6   05FCN   4M   06/05

First printing June 2005.

This appendix is not current and is of historical significance only.

ACKNOWLEDGMENTS

Work Group Members
Peggy S. Matteson, PhD, RN, FCN, *Chair*
Rev. Sheryl S. Cross, MSN, MDiv, RN, FCN
Dianne Foglesong, MSN, RN, FCN
Amy Hickman, BS, RN,
Lynne Roy, MSN, RN, FCN
Nancy L. Rago Durbin, MA, MS, RNC, FCN
Roberta Schweitzer, PhD, RN, FCN
Sonja Simpson, MSN, RN, HNC, FCN
Sybil D. Smith, PhD, RN, FCN
Susan L. Ward PhD, RN, FCN

ANA Staff
Carol Bickford, PhD, RN, BC – Content editor
Yvonne Humes, MSA – Project coordinator
Winifred Carson, JD – Legal counsel

This appendix is not current and is of historical significance only.

CONTENTS

This appendix is not current and is of historical significance only.

This appendix is not current and is of historical significance only.

INTRODUCTION

There have been dramatic changes in health care and the profession of nursing during the past decade. *Nursing: Scope and Standards of Practice* (ANA 2004) provided the framework and direction for review and revision of this scope and standards of practice. The purpose of this document is to describe the specialty practice of faith community nursing and to provide faith community nurses, the nursing profession, other healthcare providers, spiritual leaders, employers, insurers, and their patients with an understanding of the unique scope of knowledge and the standards of care and professional performance expected of a faith community nurse (FCN).

Function of the Scope of Practice Statement of Faith Community Nursing

The scope of practice statement describes the *who, what, where, when, why,* and *how* of the practice of faith community nursing. The answers to these questions provide a complete picture of the practice, its boundaries, and its membership.

Nursing: Scope and Standards of Practice (ANA 2004*)* applies to all professional registered nurses engaged in practice, regardless of specialty, practice setting, or educational preparation. With *Code of Ethics for Nurses with Interpretive Statements* (ANA 2001*)* and *Nursing's Social Policy Statement* (ANA 2003), it forms the foundation of practice for all registered nurses. The scope of faith community nursing practice is specific to this specialty, but builds on the scope of care expected of all registered nurses.

Function of the Standards of Faith Community Nursing

"Standards are authoritative statements by which the nursing profession describes the responsibilities for which its practitioners are accountable. Consequently, standards reflect the values and priorities of the profession. Standards provide direction for professional nursing practice and a framework for evaluation of this practice. Written in measurable terms, these standards define the nursing profession's accountability to the public and the outcomes for which registered nurses are responsible" (ANA 2004, 1). The standards of faith community nursing practice are specific to this specialty, but build on the standards of care expected of all registered nurses.

This appendix is not current and is of historical significance only.

Development of *Faith Community Nursing: Scope and Standards of Practice*

As the professional organization for all registered nurses, the American Nurses Association (ANA) has assumed the responsibility for developing generic scope and standards that apply to the practice of all professional nurses. *Nursing: Scope and Standards of Practice* (ANA 2004) describes what nursing is, what nurses do, and the responsibilities for which they are accountable.

Health Ministries Association (HMA), the professional membership organization for nurses in this specialty, and ANA collaborated in the development and publication of *Scope and Standards of Parish Nursing Practice* in 1998. With the publication of the new Foundation of Nursing documents, all specialty scope and standards are now being revised. For continuity and consistency, *Nursing: Scope and Standards of Practice* (ANA 2004) was used as the template when developing this document.

During 2003 and early 2004, HMA requested volunteers to serve on a working group to review and revise the scope and standards. Ten practicing nurses representing different parts of the country and various roles in this specialty practice convened and started work in February 2004. In August a draft was posted on the HMA web site for six weeks of public review. Hard copies of the document were also distributed on request. More than 200 responses were received and carefully considered. As a result, this document provides a national perspective on the current practice of this evolving specialty of faith community nursing.

Summary

These standards and scope of practice for faith community nursing reflect the commitment of Health Ministries Association, Inc., to work with American Nurses Association to promote understanding of faith community nursing as a specialized practice in the multidisciplinary practice arena of diverse faith communities. HMA is the national professional organization representing faith community nurses and others working in the expanding faith community arena.

As the diversity of participating faith communities expands in rural areas, towns, and cities, the difficulty in finding all-inclusive terminology to describe the beliefs and practices that have evolved from dissimilar traditions becomes more apparent. Terms used in this document indicate an effort to include all faith traditions, not to promote any one faith tradition.

This appendix is not current and is of historical significance only.

Faith Community Nursing: Scope and Standards of Practice reflects current faith community nursing practice from a national perspective, the professional and ethical standards of the nursing profession, and the legal scope and standards of professional nursing practice. They are dynamic and subject to testing and change.

This appendix is not current and is of historical significance only.

STANDARDS OF FAITH COMMUNITY NURSING PRACTICE: STANDARDS OF PRACTICE

STANDARD 1. ASSESSMENT

The faith community nurse collects comprehensive data pertinent to the patient's wholistic health or the situation.

STANDARD 2. DIAGNOSIS

The faith community nurse analyzes the wholistic assessment data to determine the diagnoses or issues.

STANDARD 3. OUTCOMES IDENTIFICATION

The faith community nurse identifies expected outcomes for a plan individualized to the patient or the situation.

STANDARD 4. PLANNING

The faith community nurse develops a plan that prescribes strategies and alternatives to attain expected outcomes for individuals, groups, or the faith community as a whole.

STANDARD 5. IMPLEMENTATION

The faith community nurse implements the specified plan.

STANDARD 5A: COORDINATION OF CARE

The faith community nurse coordinates care delivery.

STANDARD 5B: HEALTH TEACHING AND HEALTH PROMOTION

The faith community nurse employs strategies to promote wholistic health, wellness, and a safe environment.

STANDARD 5C: CONSULTATION

The faith community nurse provides consultation to facilitate understanding and influence the specified plan of care, enhance the abilities of others, and effect change.

STANDARD 5D: PRESCRIPTIVE AUTHORITY AND TREATMENT

(Optional for appropriately prepared APRN)
The advanced practice registered nurse, faith community nurse uses prescriptive authority, procedures, referrals, treatments, and therapies in accordance with state and federal laws and regulations.

STANDARD 6. EVALUATION

The faith community nurse evaluates progress toward attainment of outcomes.

This appendix is not current and is of historical significance only.

Standards of Faith Community Nursing Practice: Standards of Professional Performance

Standard 7. Quality of Practice

The faith community nurse systematically enhances the quality and effectiveness of faith community nursing practice.

Standard 8. Education

The faith community nurse attains knowledge and competency that reflects current nursing practice.

Standard 9. Professional Practice Evaluation

The faith community nurse evaluates one's own nursing practice in relation to professional practice standards and guidelines, relevant statutes, rules, and regulations.

Standard 10. Collegiality

The faith community nurse interacts with and contributes to the professional development of peers and colleagues.

Standard 11. Collaboration

The faith community nurse collaborates with the patient, spiritual leaders, members of the faith community, and others in the conduct of this specialized nursing practice.

Standard 12. Ethics

The faith community nurse integrates ethical provisions in all areas of practice.

Standard 13. Research

The faith community nurse integrates research findings into practice.

Standard 14. Resource Utilization

The faith community nurse considers factors related to safety, effectiveness, cost, and impact on practice in the planning and delivery of nursing services.

Standard 15. Leadership

The faith community nurse provides leadership in the professional practice setting and the profession.

This appendix is not current and is of historical significance only.

SCOPE OF FAITH COMMUNITY NURSING PRACTICE

Definition and Overview of Faith Community Nursing

Faith community nursing is the specialized practice of professional nursing that focuses on the intentional care of the spirit as part of the process of promoting wholistic health and preventing or minimizing illness in a faith community.

The faith community nurse (FCN) is knowledgeable in two areas—professional nursing and spiritual care. As a member of the staff providing spiritual care in the faith community, the goal of an FCN is the protection, promotion, and optimization of health and abilities; prevention of illness and injury; and responding to suffering in the context of the values, beliefs, and practices of a faith community such as a church, congregation, parish, synagogue, temple, or mosque.

The FCN uses the nursing process to address the spiritual, physical, mental, and social health of the patient. The term *patient* may refer to the faith community as a whole, or groups, families, and individuals in the faith community. Residents from the vicinity of the faith community may also seek the services of the FCN.

With an intentional focus on spiritual health, the FCN primarily uses the nursing interventions of education, counseling, advocacy, referral, utilizing resources available to the faith community, and training and supervising volunteers from the faith community. As an actively licensed registered nurse, the FCN provides nursing care based on professional and legal expectations, education, professional experience, the needs of the patient population, and the position as defined in the faith community. The FCN collaborates with other nursing specialties such as community health, hospice, rehabilitation, home health, acute care, and critical care in other aspects of nursing care for the faith community and its members.

This document—in conjunction with *Nursing's Social Policy Statement* (ANA 2003); *Nursing: Scope and Standards of Practice* (ANA 2004); *Code of Ethics for Nurses with Interpretive Statements* (ANA 2001); and the laws, statutes, and regulations related to nursing practice for their state, commonwealth, or territory—delineates the professional responsibilities of an FCN.

This appendix is not current and is of historical significance only.

Evolution of Faith Community Nursing

Nursing has its historical roots in the link between faith and healing in the ancient traditions of most major religions. This relationship evolved over time, influenced by cultural, political, social, and economic events. Religious groups founded hospitals to provide care to vulnerable populations such as the poor, immigrant, and homeless, and during the last century developed schools of nursing.

In 1979, Rev. Dr. Granger Westberg received grant funding to create Wholistic Health Centers in Christian congregations, staffed by a treatment/healing team comprised of a doctor, a nurse, a social worker, and a pastoral counselor. The nurses in these centers were referred to as "parish nurses." Since then various other faith communities have established programs of health and healing led by a registered nurse. The word "parish" in *parish nurse* is not acceptable in all faith traditions, so faith communities have created different titles for this specialized nursing role. To have one name inclusive of all faith traditions and to accurately label the location and focus of practice, the specialty practice described in this document is titled "faith community nursing." In a given setting, the faith community nurse may still be referred to as a *parish nurse, congregational nurse, health ministry nurse, crescent nurse,* or *health and wellness nurse.*

Westberg used the term "wholistic health" to define a whole or completely integrated approach to health and health care that integrates the physical and spiritual aspects of the whole person. The principles of wholistic health arose from the understanding that human beings strive for wholeness in relationship to their God, themselves, their families, and the society in which they live. Based on its historic meaning, then, *wholistic* is the preferred spelling when referring to the health care provided by faith community nurses.

Nurse-led programs within and beyond Judeo-Christian faith communities continue to grow and evolve. The common expectation across faith traditions is that the professional registered nurse functioning as an FCN possesses a depth of understanding of the faith community's traditions, as well as competence as a registered nurse using the nursing process so that the nursing care integrates care of the spirit with that of the body and mind.

Assumptions of Faith Community Nursing

These five assumptions underlie faith community nursing:

- Health and illness are human experiences.
- Health is the integration of the spiritual, physical, psychological, and social aspects of the patient promoting a sense of harmony with self, others, the environment, and a higher power.

This appendix is not current and is of historical significance only.

- Health may be experienced in the presence of disease or injury.

- The presence of illness does not preclude health nor does optimal health preclude illness.

- Healing is the process of integrating the body, mind, and spirit to create wholeness, health, and a sense of well-being, even when the patient's illness is not cured.

Focusing on Spiritual Care in the Art of Nursing

Nurses have long observed that when illness or brokenness occurs, patients—whether individually or with their family or friends—may turn to their source of spiritual strength for reassurance, support, and healing. *Nursing: Scope and Standards of Practice* (ANA 2004) reaffirms that spiritual care is a part of all nursing practice. The primary focus of the FCN is the intentional care of the spirit, differentiating this specialty practice from the general practice of a registered nurse. Within this specialized knowledge base, each FCN will demonstrate competence on a continuum from novice to expert.

A variety of tools for spiritual assessment have been developed and tested for reliability and validity. These tools, varying from simple screening to in-depth assessments, are increasingly used in nursing practice. Since the use of spiritual assessment tools has not been generally taught to providers from other disciplines, the FCN may provide leadership to the staff in the selection and application of assessment tools.

After analyzing the assessment data, the FCN selects the nursing diagnoses to describe actual or potential needs of the patient, including spiritual needs. These diagnoses then provide the basis for nursing interventions to achieve the outcomes for which the nurse is accountable. Examples of nursing diagnoses accepted by the North American Nursing Diagnosis Association (NANDA) related specifically to spiritual care are Spiritual Distress, Risk for Spiritual Distress, and Readiness for Spiritual Well-being (NANDA 2005).

Treatment may or may not cure an affliction. However, it is still possible through care of the spirit for a person to be healed even if a cure—physical restoration—does not occur. A patient may be dying from cancer, but if a broken relationship between family members has been reconciled or the patient is at peace with the circumstances, this may be considered healing.

Assault, betrayal, accident, or death of a member can affect an entire faith community. Members of all ages may manifest anger, grief, anxiety, fear, and spiritual or physical pain in varying degrees. An FCN's response to such an event is complex. Beyond identifying and meeting the needs of individuals and families, the FCN treats the whole faith community as a patient. Assessment focuses on identifying the educational and supportive needs of

This appendix is not current and is of historical significance only.

the whole faith community. Interventions occur at three different levels: community, family or group, and individual.

From a less dramatic but equally important perspective, the FCN will address a variety of issues that threaten the wholistic health of participants in the faith community:

- Individuals or families may lack food, shelter, transportation, income, or health care.

- Victims of domestic violence or other forms of abuse may seek solace or sanctuary.

- Adult children of aging parents may seek guidance in talking with or determining the appropriate living situation for a parent, and ongoing assistance from the faith community.

To respond to these and other situations wholistically, an FCN draws on professional skills that integrate spiritual care and nursing care, and the resources of individuals and groups both within and beyond the faith community to provide a wholistic response. Some patients will require support of basic needs so that they have the time and space to reflect on spiritual issues; for others, spiritual care will be the direct response.

The form that spiritual care takes will depend upon the beliefs and practices of the faith community; the desire of the faith community, the group, or the individual; the skills of the faith community nurse; and the collaboration of other staff members and volunteers.

Educational Preparation for Faith Community Nursing

The faith community nurse bridges two disciplines and thus must be prepared in and responsible to both. This document provides a complete picture of the specialty practice and its boundaries and membership from the perspective of the nursing profession; each faith group may provide additional stipulations and requirements. There are designations in the specialty that indicate the level of education achieved.

Appropriate and effective practice as an FCN requires the ability to integrate current nursing, behavioral, environmental, and spiritual knowledge with the unique spiritual beliefs and practices of the faith community into a program of wholistic nursing care. This is necessary no matter what level of education the nurse has achieved. With education, mentoring, and a collaborative practice site, an FCN may progress from novice to expert in this specialty practice.

This appendix is not current and is of historical significance only.

Faith Community Nurse

The preferred minimum preparation for a registered nurse or advanced practice registered nurse entering the specialty of faith community nursing includes:

- A baccalaureate or higher degree in nursing with academic preparation in community nursing,

- Experience as a registered nurse using the nursing process,

- Knowledge of the healthcare assets of the community,

- Specialized knowledge of the spiritual beliefs and practices of the faith community, and

- Specialized knowledge and skills to enable implementation of *Faith Community Nursing: Scope and Standards of Practice.*

Currently, the education of all nursing students preparing for the national examination for RN licensure includes basic content on spiritual care. In addition, an increasing number of undergraduate students during their community health courses participate in clinical experiences with faith community nurses. However, because of the intentional focus on spiritual care by the faith community nurse, this educational exposure is not adequate preparation for assuming the specialty role of an FCN.

A registered nurse may prepare for the specialty of faith community nursing in one of several ways. Educational offerings range from continuing education programs with extensive contact hours to baccalaureate and graduate level nursing courses. Some colleges that specialize in religious education also offer relevant courses or programs of study. Collaboration between disciplines has also led to the offering of dual master's degrees in nursing and theology or health ministry. Registered nurses may also participate in online education with or without academic credit. Faith communities understand, support, and often fund continuing education of FCNs to enhance their ability to provide spiritual care, knowing that this directly benefits their own programs.

Specialty certification programs generally require psychometrically sound and legally defensible certification examinations. These are possible only with sufficient applicants and adequate financial resources. At this time, specialty certification in faith community nursing is not available. Because faith community nurses work in churches, synagogues, temples, mosques, and other faith community settings and not in healthcare facilities, certification currently has little bearing on the decision of a committee or board in a faith community to engage the professional services of an FCN. Other models for specialty certification, such as professional portfolios, are being explored.

This appendix is not current and is of historical significance only.

Advanced Practice Registered Nurse

Increasing numbers of advanced practice registered nurses (APRNs: nurse practitioners and clinical nurse specialists) are acquiring the additional specialized education that prepares them for practice as a faith community nurse. By definition, an advanced practice registered nurse has a master's or doctoral degree that prepares the nurse to be a clinical expert in evidence-based nursing practice. An APRN, FCN has earned the designation as either a clinical nurse specialist or a nurse practitioner, and has also prepared for the role of an FCN. The APRN, FCN integrates theoretical and evidence-based knowledge from graduate nursing education with the specialized education of an FCN regarding the structure, spiritual beliefs, and practices of the faith group. These advanced practice nurses are held to a higher standard of expertise when providing nursing care.

The APRN, FCN designs, implements, and evaluates both population-specific and patient-specific programs of wholistic care for the faith community. An APRN, FCN provides leadership in advancing this specialty nursing practice to achieve quality and cost-effective wholistic patient outcomes, and leads multidisciplinary groups in designing and implementing innovative alternative solutions to problems and patient issues essential to spiritual health and well-being.

In addition to providing nursing care, the APRN, FCN influences nursing care outcomes by serving as an advocate, consultant, or researcher in the specialty area; providing expert consultation for spiritual leaders and other healthcare providers; and by identifying and facilitating improvements in wholistic health care.

Laws, regulations, and rules concerning certification as an advanced practice nurse are issued by state licensing or regulatory boards, and vary among states. Each FCN seeking to attain the APRN designation must meet the requirements of the jurisdiction of practice as well as the standards of practice set forth in this document.

Additional Designations

National leaders of faith groups that recognize the importance of integrating this specialty nursing practice into faith communities have developed mechanisms for mentoring and providing informal and formal education in concepts of spiritual beliefs, practices, and rituals. When such facilities are available within the faith group, the FCN may work with the leadership of the faith community to meet the educational and practice requirements to earn formal designation as a spiritual leader.

This appendix is not current and is of historical significance only.

Faith groups have different ways of designating or titling individuals who have attained an advanced level of preparation and often undergone examination to determine fitness for providing spiritual care. The FCN who achieves the requirements defined by the faith group in which they are practicing may then be given a title by the faith community indicating their achievement. Examples of such titles are *Deacon, Minister of Health,* or *Pastoral Associate.* Titles such as these have a specialized meaning within the faith community served.

Settings for Practice in Faith Community Nursing

An FCN serves as a member of the multidisciplinary staff of a faith community, providing care to the faith community as a whole as well as to member groups and individuals. The FCN is the sole healthcare provider responsible for practice in this non-healthcare setting, although others from the faith community assist the FCN.

Most encounters with patients are initiated within the buildings and programs of the faith community. Participants in the various activities of the faith community, such as worship, education, special interest or support groups, programs for spiritual growth or renewal, and support services such as soup kitchens, may seek the services of the FCN.

A community of faith may be composed of people of all ages. The members may also offer a range of physical, emotional, and cognitive development. When an individual, family, group, or the faith community as a whole experiences or desires a change in their level of physical, mental, social, environmental, or spiritual well-being, or when maintaining their current level of well-being requires nursing action, an FCN collaborates with them to develop a plan of care that incorporates communal and individual spiritual beliefs and practices.

The FCN monitors environmental and safety issues of the facilities and chooses appropriate responses in collaboration with the leadership of the faith community. The FCN also manages physical and mental health issues, including the high levels of stress of spiritual leaders, other staff members, or faith community volunteers, with interventions that encompass spiritual support, health promotion, illness prevention, and disease management.

The needs and desires of individual members of the faith community may require that the FCN visit members in the hospital or a hospice, in private homes or residential facilities, or accompany patients as they use health services in the community. During these encounters the FCN may also intervene with spiritual care and provide a supportive, healing presence for both the patient and loved ones.

This appendix is not current and is of historical significance only.

The size, concerns, and expectations of the faith community will determine the expected role of an FCN. As a staff member, the FCN is most often supported and guided by a committee of faith community members and assisted by lay volunteers. With education and supervision provided by the FCN, these volunteers may assume tasks that family members would do for each other if they were available. This type of supportive team, led by the FCN, can increase safety and comfort during hospital discharge transitions and provide patients with comprehensive support once home, helping them to recuperate more easily or to achieve peace before death.

Continued Commitment to the Profession

The specialty practice of faith community nursing is relatively new, and requires that each FCN educate other healthcare providers and the general public concerning the benefits of this nursing care. An faith community nurse may participate with colleagues in the community, such as an FNC group or a clergy association, to develop collaborative efforts throughout the community.

The FCN commits to lifelong learning in both nursing and the beliefs and practices of the faith community. There are numerous opportunities for personal and professional growth both in and beyond the community. Major denominations support both programs and professional development. The professional organization for faith community nurses, the Health Ministries Association, provides opportunities for networking and ongoing education both in the specialty as well as with other disciplines. A variety of educational institutions and resource centers are also available around the country or online.

While the FCN may be the only healthcare provider in the faith community, the best practice cannot be provided in isolation. Personal and professional support, education opportunities, and resources are available. Accessing these will improve both the care provided to the faith community and the progress of the specialty.

Research

Research conducted at the National Institutes of Health and academic institutions has established a relationship between spiritual practices and health, thereby expanding the knowledge base for the specialty of faith community nursing. Findings from a variety of non-nursing disciplines provide understanding of the strong connection between spiritual well-being, participation in religious practices, and wholistic health. Involvement in a faith community provides health benefits through social support, a social identity, and a sense of power beyond one's self. Religious and spiritual practices such

This appendix is not current and is of historical significance only.

as meditation, prayer, and touch are reported to lengthen life, improve the quality of life, and improve health outcomes by enhancing psychological, physical, and spiritual well-being. Research reports may be found in the nursing literature and publications of other health professionals, as well as the professional literature focused on health ministry, chaplaincy, theology, spirituality, spiritual care, and pastoral care.

Research by faith community nurses to evaluate the benefits of this specialty practice is slowly emerging. Funding would enhance efforts to establish programs of collaborative research between practicing faith community nurses and nurse researchers that could validate and promote the wholistic health benefits of this nursing specialty in the multidisciplinary environment. Confirmation of positive outcomes would be a major influence in funding further research and positions for faith community nurses.

Professional Trends and Issues

Since 1998, when faith community nursing was formally recognized as a specialty practice, there has been tremendous growth in both professional knowledge and the number of faith communities seeking such services. With this growth, several issues have become more apparent:

- *What to call nurse providers so that the title is understood across various faith groups.* This issue has been addressed with the adoption of an all-encompassing title for this specialty. Sensitivity to the desires of individual faith communities to maintain their own internal title has also been considered. Just as each community calls their spiritual leader by their own title, such as rabbi, pastor, minister, teacher, they may also call the FCN by the title they choose. However, selection of an internal title different than faith community nurse does not relieve that registered nurse from fulfilling the expectations set forth in this document.

- *Identifying the preparation needed for this evolving specialty practice.* This discussion is ongoing. When educational resources for this specialty were difficult to obtain, nurses had minimal opportunities. With the clarification of minimum standards and an increasing awareness by nurse educators and practicing nurses of the requirements for this specialty practice, both educational expectations and opportunities are increasing at all levels of nursing education.

- *Engaging other practice disciplines and faith communities in accepting this specialty nursing practice.* As the number and professional activities of faith community nurses increase, so too does the recognition of these specialists by other disciplines. Faith community nurses are vital partners in advancing the nation's health initiatives such as Healthy People 2010 to increase the quality and years of healthy life and eliminate health

This appendix is not current and is of historical significance only.

disparities. As members of faith communities experience the benefit of care from an FCN and share their experiences with others, the demand for these services will increase.

- *Creation of paid positions so that more professional nurses may choose to enter the specialty.* Financial compensation for providing faith community nursing services is a complex subject familiar to those who know the history of compensation in professional nursing. In this case, the issue is complicated by three major factors:
  - A lack of financial resources in many faith communities for an expansion of services,
  - A faith community's tradition of donating time and expertise to care for each other, and
  - Difficulty in obtaining objective data that demonstrates the positive health affects and benefits of faith community nursing so that external funding will be more available.

As with any complex issue, addressing this situation will be a multifaceted process. Some faith community nurses choose to provide care part- or full-time, at low financial compensation if any, as part of their gift to the faith community. Others provide care so that they may demonstrate the value of this specialty practice and collect data to support the hiring of a faith community nurse for that community of faith. Some nurses, taking a broader perspective, work within faith community organizations to increase recognition of this specialty nursing practice as a form of spiritual leadership worthy of financial support. Still others are encouraging healthcare organizations and facilities to provide financial support of an FCN in faith communities. Given the varied dynamics of individual communities of faith, there is no one solution.

This document delineates the professional expectations associated with this specialty practice. When it is considered in conjunction with *Nursing's Social Policy Statement* (ANA 2003), *Nursing: Scope and Standards of Practice* (ANA 2004), and *Code of Ethics for Nurses with Interpretive Statements* (ANA 2001), the professional nurse receives clear guidance in the requirements for preparation and practice that best serve the public's health and the nursing profession.

This appendix is not current and is of historical significance only.

Standards of Faith Community Nursing Practice
Standards of Practice

Standard 1. Assessment

The faith community nurse collects comprehensive data pertinent to the patient's wholistic health or the situation.

Measurement Criteria:

The faith community nurse:

- Prioritizes data collection activities based on the patient's immediate condition, or the anticipated needs of the patient or situation.

- Collects wholistic data in a systematic and ongoing process, with a particular emphasis on spiritual beliefs and practices.

- Involves the patient, family, group, spiritual leader, other healthcare providers, and others, as appropriate, in wholistic data collection.

- Uses appropriate evidence-based assessment techniques and instruments in collecting pertinent data as a basis for wholistic care.

- Uses analytical models and problem-solving tools.

- Synthesizes available data, information, and knowledge relevant to the situation to identify patterns and variances in individuals, families, groups, or the faith community as a whole.

- Documents and stores relevant data in a retrievable format that is both confidential and secure.

Additional Measurement Criteria for the Advanced Practice Registered Nurse, Faith Community Nurse:

The advanced practice registered nurse, faith community nurse:

- Interprets results from diagnostic tests relevant to the wholistic assessment of the patient's current status.

This appendix is not current and is of historical significance only.

Standard 2. Diagnosis

The faith community nurse analyzes the wholistic assessment data to determine the diagnoses or issues.

Measurement Criteria:

The faith community nurse:

- Derives the diagnoses or issues based on wholistic assessment data.

- Identifies strengths that enhance health and spiritual well-being.

- Identifies actual, perceived, or potential threats to health and spiritual well-being.

- Validates the diagnoses or issues with the patient, family, spiritual leader, and other healthcare providers, when possible and appropriate.

- Documents diagnoses in a manner that facilitates the determination of the expected outcomes and plan.

Additional Measurement Criteria for the Advanced Practice Registered Nurse, Faith Community Nurse:

The advanced practice registered nurse, faith community nurse:

- Systematically compares and contrasts assessment data with normal and abnormal variations and developmental events in formulating a differential diagnosis.

- Utilizes complex data and information obtained during interview, wholistic assessment, and diagnostic procedures in identifying diagnoses.

- Assists registered nurses in developing and maintaining competency in the diagnostic process.

This appendix is not current and is of historical significance only.

STANDARD 3. OUTCOMES IDENTIFICATION

The faith community nurse identifies expected outcomes for a plan individualized to the patient or the situation.

Measurement Criteria:

The faith community nurse:

- Involves the patient, spiritual leaders, and healthcare providers in formulating expected outcomes when possible and as appropriate.

- Derives culturally and spiritually appropriate expected outcomes from the identified diagnoses.

- Considers spiritual beliefs and practices, associated benefits, costs, risks, current scientific evidence, and clinical expertise when formulating expected outcomes.

- Defines expected outcomes in terms of the patient, patient values, faith beliefs and practices, ethical considerations, family perspectives, cultural practices, environment, or situation with such considerations as associated benefits, risks, and costs, and current scientific evidence.

- Develops expected outcomes that focus on patients attaining, maintaining, or regaining health or healing, with a particular emphasis on patient-identified spiritual well-being.

- Identifies expected outcomes that incorporate spiritual beliefs and practices with current scientific evidence and are achievable through implementation of evidence-based practices.

- Includes a realistic time estimate for attainment of expected outcomes.

- Develops in a collaborative process expected outcomes that provide direction for continuity of care.

- Modifies expected outcomes based on changes in the desires of the patient, the status of the patient, or evaluation of the situation.

- Documents expected outcomes as measurable goals.

Continued ▸

This appendix is not current and is of historical significance only.

Additional Measurement Criteria for the Advanced Practice Registered Nurse, Faith Community Nurse:

The advanced practice registered nurse, faith community nurse:

- Identifies expected outcomes that incorporate patient satisfaction with care and quality of life, cost and clinical effectiveness, and continuity and consistency between patient's spiritual beliefs and healthcare interventions.

- Supports the use of clinical and spiritual guidelines linked to positive patient outcomes of wholistic health and healing.

This appendix is not current and is of historical significance only.

STANDARD 4. PLANNING

The faith community nurse develops a plan that prescribes strategies and alternatives to attain expected outcomes for individuals, groups, or the faith community as a whole.

Measurement Criteria:

The faith community nurse:

- Develops an individualized plan considering patient characteristics, spiritual beliefs and practices, and the situation.

- Develops the plan in conjunction with the patient, spiritual leaders, and others, as appropriate.

- Includes strategies in the plan that address each of the identified diagnoses or issues, which may include strategies for promotion and restoration of health, spiritual enhancement, and prevention of illness, injury, and disease.

- Integrates current trends and research affecting care in the planning process.

- Defines the plan to reflect current statutes, rules, regulations, and standards.

- Considers the economic impact of the plan and how the faith community and local community resources might be of assistance.

- Establishes the priorities in the plan with the patient, and others, as appropriate.

- Participates in the design and development of multidisciplinary and interdisciplinary processes to address the situation or issue.

- Incorporates an implementation pathway or realistic timeline in the plan.

- Provides for continuity of care and appropriate communication in the plan.

- Uses recognized terminology or standardized language to document the plan.

- Communicates the plan, with the consent of the patient, to others involved in providing care.

Continued ▶

- Supports the integration of the resources of the faith community to enhance and complete the patient's decision-making processes.

- Utilizes the plan to provide direction to other members of the healthcare team.

- Contributes to the development and continuous improvement of the organizational systems of the faith community that support the planning process.

Additional Measurement Criteria for the Advanced Practice Registered Nurse, Faith Community Nurse:

The advanced practice registered nurse, faith community nurse:

- Identifies assessment, diagnostic strategies, and therapeutic interventions in the plan that reflect current evidence, including data, research, literature, and expert nursing knowledge to enhance wholistic health.

- Selects or designs strategies to meet the multifaceted wholistic needs of complex patients.

- Includes the synthesis of patients' values and spiritual beliefs regarding nursing and medical therapies in the plan.

This appendix is not current and is of historical significance only.

STANDARD 5. IMPLEMENTATION

The faith community nurse implements the specified plan.

Measurement Criteria:

The faith community nurse:

- Collaborates with the patient and support system to implement the plan in a safe and timely manner.

- Collaborates with and empowers patients to enhance their spiritual well-being and healthy behaviors, reduce the occurrence of illness, modify health risk behaviors, and adapt to chronic changes in health status.

- Documents implementation and any modifications, including changes or omissions, of the specified plan.

- Utilizes evidence-based interventions and treatments specific to the diagnosis or issue.

- Utilizes resources and systems in the faith community and the community in which it is located to implement the plan.

- Collaborates with spiritual leaders, faith community volunteers, caregivers, nursing colleagues, and others to implement the plan.

- Fosters organizational systems and programs in the faith community that support implementation of the plan.

Additional Measurement Criteria for the Advanced Practice Registered Nurse, Faith Community Nurse:

The advanced practice registered nurse, faith community nurse:

- Develops and utilizes systems in the faith community and other community resources when necessary to implement the plan.

- Supports the development of multidisciplinary collaboration to implement the plan.

- Incorporates new knowledge and strategies to initiate change in faith community nursing care practices if desired outcomes are not achieved.

This appendix is not current and is of historical significance only.

STANDARD 5A: COORDINATION OF CARE

The faith community nurse coordinates care delivery.

Measurement Criteria:

The faith community nurse:

- Coordinates implementation of the plan of care.
- Advocates for the patient's desired plan of care with other professionals and healthcare agencies.
- Documents the coordination of care in a secure and retrievable format.

Additional Measurement Criteria for the Advanced Practice Registered Nurse, Faith Community Nurse:

The advanced practice registered nurse, faith community nurse:

- Provides leadership in the coordination of multidisciplinary health care for integrated delivery of patient care services for members of a faith community.
- Synthesizes data and information to prescribe necessary system and community support measures, including environmental modifications, spiritual support, and faith-based interventions.
- Coordinates system and community resources that enhance delivery of care across continuums.

This appendix is not current and is of historical significance only.

STANDARD 5B: HEALTH TEACHING AND HEALTH PROMOTION

The faith community nurse employs strategies to promote wholistic health, wellness, and a safe environment.

Measurement Criteria:

The faith community nurse:

- Teaches activities that strengthen the body–mind–spirit connection such as meditation, prayer, and guided imagery.

- Facilitates educational programs for individuals or groups that address such topics as spiritual practices for health and healing, healthy lifestyles, risk-reducing behaviors, developmental needs, activities of daily living, and self-care.

- Uses health promotion and health teaching methods appropriate to the situation, the faith community, and the patient's spiritual beliefs and practices, developmental level, learning needs, readiness, ability to learn, language or communication preference, and culture.

- Evaluates health information resources for use in faith community nursing for accuracy, readability, and comprehensibility by patients, and compatibility with patients' spiritual beliefs and practices.

- Seeks ongoing opportunities for feedback and evaluation of the effectiveness of the strategies used.

Additional Measurement Criteria for the Advanced Practice Registered Nurse, Faith Community Nurse:

The advanced practice registered nurse, faith community nurse:

- Synthesizes empirical evidence on spiritual practices, risk behaviors, learning theories, behavioral change theories, motivational theories, epidemiology, and other related theories and frameworks when designing wholistic health information and patient education.

- Designs health information and patient education appropriate to the patient's spiritual beliefs and practices, cultural values and beliefs, developmental level, learning needs, readiness to learn, and readiness to experience new spiritual practices.

- Evaluates health information resources, such as the Internet, for accuracy, readability, and comprehensibility to help patients access quality health information that is compatible with their spiritual beliefs and practices.

STANDARD 5C: CONSULTATION

The faith community nurse provides consultation to facilitate understanding and influence the specified plan of care, enhance the abilities of others, and effect change.

Measurement Criteria:

The faith community nurse:

- Synthesizes information on beliefs and practices of the faith community when providing consultation.

- Facilitates the effectiveness of a consultation by involving the patient in the decision-making process and negotiation of role responsibilities.

Additional Measurement Criteria for the Advanced Practice Registered Nurse, Faith Community Nurse:

The advanced practice registered nurse, faith community nurse:

- Synthesizes spiritual practices, organizational structure and beliefs of the faith group, clinical data, theoretical frameworks, and evidence when providing consultation.

- Facilitates the effectiveness of a consultation by involving the patient or their designee in decision-making and negotiating role responsibilities for each member of the faith community team.

This appendix is not current and is of historical significance only.

Standard 5d: Prescriptive Authority and Treatment

(Optional for appropriately prepared APRN)

The advanced practice registered nurse, faith community nurse uses prescriptive authority, procedures, referrals, treatments, and therapies in accordance with state and federal laws and regulations.

Measurement Criteria for the Advanced Practice Registered Nurse, Faith Community Nurse:

The advanced practice registered nurse, faith community nurse:

- Prescribes evidence-based treatments, therapies, and procedures, considering the patient's comprehensive healthcare needs and their spiritual needs, beliefs, and practices.

- Prescribes therapies, including those that strengthen the body–mind–spirit connection such as meditation, prayer, guided imagery, and various rituals of worship.

- Prescribes pharmacological agents based on a current knowledge of pharmacology and physiology.

- Prescribes specific pharmacological agents and treatments based on clinical indicators, the patient's status and needs, and the results of diagnostic assessments and laboratory tests.

- Evaluates therapeutic and potential adverse effects of pharmacological and non-pharmacological treatments.

- Provides patients with information about intended effects and potential adverse effects of proposed prescriptive therapies.

- Provides information about costs, and complementary and alternative treatments and procedures, as appropriate.

This appendix is not current and is of historical significance only.

Standard 6. Evaluation

The faith community nurse evaluates progress toward attainment of outcomes.

Measurement Criteria:

The faith community nurse:

- Conducts a wholistic, systematic, ongoing, and criterion-based evaluation of the outcomes in relation to the structures and processes described by the plan and the indicated timeline.

- Includes the patient and others involved in the care or situation in the evaluative process.

- Evaluates the effectiveness of the planned strategies in relation to patient responses and attainment of expected outcomes.

- Documents the results of the evaluation, including results from the faith or spiritual realm.

- Uses ongoing assessment data to revise the diagnoses, the outcomes, the plan, and the implementation as needed.

- Disseminates the results to the patient and others involved in the care or situation, as appropriate, in accordance with state and federal laws and regulations.

- Uses the results of the evaluation analyses to make or recommend process or program changes in the faith community, as appropriate, to improve the provision and outcomes of care.

Additional Measurement Criteria for the Advanced Practice Registered Nurse, Faith Community Nurse:

The advanced practice registered nurse, faith community nurse:

- Evaluates the accuracy of the diagnosis and effectiveness of the interventions in relation to the patient's attainment of expected outcomes.

- Synthesizes the results of the evaluation analyses to determine the impact of the plan on the affected patients, families, groups, faith communities and institutions, collegial networks, organizations, and geopolitical communities.

- Uses the results of the evaluation analyses to increase awareness beyond the individual faith community of the wholistic health benefits and spiritual care provided through faith community nursing.

This appendix is not current and is of historical significance only.

STANDARDS OF PROFESSIONAL PERFORMANCE

STANDARD 7. QUALITY OF PRACTICE

The faith community nurse systematically enhances the quality and effectiveness of faith community nursing practice.

Measurement Criteria:

The faith community nurse:

- Obtains and maintains designation and recognition as a spiritual care provider in a faith community.

- Demonstrates quality by documenting the application of the nursing process in a responsible, accountable, and ethical manner.

- Uses the results of quality improvement activities to initiate changes in the practice of faith community nursing and in the interaction between a faith community and the healthcare delivery system.

- Uses creativity and innovation in faith community nursing practice to improve care delivery.

- Incorporates new knowledge to initiate changes in faith community nursing practice if desired outcomes are not achieved.

- Participates in quality improvement activities for faith community nursing. Such activities may include:
  - Identifying aspects of practice important for quality monitoring.
  - Using indicators developed to monitor quality and effectiveness.
  - Collecting data to monitor quality and effectiveness.
  - Analyzing quality data to identify opportunities for improving practice.
  - Formulating recommendations to improve practice or outcomes.
  - Implementing activities to enhance the quality of practice.
  - Developing, implementing, and evaluating policies, procedures, and guidelines.
  - Participating on interdisciplinary teams to evaluate clinical care or health services.
  - Participating in efforts to minimize costs and unnecessary duplication.
  - Analyzing factors related to safety, satisfaction, effectiveness, and cost–benefit options.

Continued ▶

This appendix is not current and is of historical significance only.

- Analyzing leadership and organizational systems in the faith community for barriers.
- Implementing processes to remove or decrease barriers in the leadership and organizational structure of the faith community.

Additional Measurement Criteria for the Advanced Practice Registered Nurse, Faith Community Nurse:

The advanced practice registered nurse, faith community nurse:

- Obtains and maintains official designation and recognition in the faith community as a spiritual care leader, if available.

- Designs quality improvement initiatives.

- Implements initiatives to evaluate the need for change.

- Develops indicators to monitor quality and effectiveness of faith community nursing practice.

- Evaluates the practice environment and quality of nursing care rendered in relation to existing evidence, identifying opportunities for the generation and use of research.

This appendix is not current and is of historical significance only.

STANDARD 8. EDUCATION

The faith community nurse attains knowledge and competency that reflects current nursing practice.

Measurement Criteria:

The faith community nurse:

- Participates in ongoing educational activities related to spiritual care, professional nursing practice, and related professional issues.

- Demonstrates a commitment to lifelong learning through self-reflection and inquiry to identify learning needs.

- Seeks learning experiences that reflect current practice in order to maintain knowledge, skills, and competence in all dimensions of faith community nursing.

- Acquires knowledge and skills appropriate to faith community nursing practice.

- Maintains professional records that provide evidence of competency and lifelong learning in the specialty.

- Seeks experiences and formal and independent learning activities to maintain and develop the necessary professional skills and knowledge to provide spiritual care.

- Uses current research findings and other evidence to expand knowledge and enhance role performance.

Additional Measurement Criteria for the Advanced Practice Registered Nurse, Faith Community Nurse:

The advanced practice registered nurse, faith community nurse:

- Uses current healthcare research findings and other evidence to expand clinical and professional knowledge in order to better combine two disciplines, nursing and spiritual care, into one practice role.

This appendix is not current and is of historical significance only.

STANDARD 9. PROFESSIONAL PRACTICE EVALUATION

The faith community nurse evaluates one's own nursing practice in relation to professional practice standards and guidelines, relevant statutes, rules, and regulations.

Measurement Criteria:

The faith community nurse's practice reflects the application of knowledge of current practice standards, guidelines, statutes, rules, and regulations.

The faith community nurse:

- Provides age-appropriate care in a spiritually, culturally, and ethnically sensitive manner.

- Engages in self-evaluation of practice on a regular basis, identifying areas of strength as well as areas in which professional development would be beneficial.

- Obtains informal feedback regarding spiritual care and nursing practice from patients, peers, spiritual leaders, health committee members, faith community volunteers, professional colleagues, and others.

- Participates in systematic formal review, as appropriate.

- Takes action to achieve goals identified during the evaluation process.

- Provides rationales for practice beliefs, decisions, and actions as part of the informal and formal evaluation processes.

Additional Measurement Criteria for the Advanced Practice Registered Nurse, Faith Community Nurse:

The advanced practice registered nurse, faith community nurse:

- Engages in a formal process, seeking feedback regarding the integration of advanced nursing practice and spiritual care from patients, peers, professional colleagues, and others.

This appendix is not current and is of historical significance only.

STANDARD 10. COLLEGIALITY

The faith community nurse interacts with and contributes to the professional development of peers and colleagues.

Measurement Criteria:

The faith community nurse:

- Shares knowledge and skills with peers and colleagues as evidenced by activities such as patient care conferences with spiritual leaders and other healthcare providers and presentations at formal or informal meetings.

- Provides peers with feedback regarding their practice and role performance.

- Interacts with peers and colleagues to enhance one's own professional faith community nursing practice, spiritual development, and role performance.

- Maintains compassionate and caring relationships with peers and colleagues.

- Contributes to an environment that is conducive to the education of colleagues concerning the relationship between spiritual care and wholistic health.

- Contributes to a supportive, healthy, spirit-filled work environment.

- Develops a plan for ongoing spiritual care and support of wholistic health of self and colleagues.

- Participates with colleagues to directly or indirectly advance wholistic health services and spiritual well-being in faith communities.

- Mentors other faith community nurses and colleagues as appropriate.

Additional Measurement Criteria for the Advanced Practice Registered Nurse, Faith Community Nurse:

The advanced practice registered nurse, faith community nurse:

- Models expert practice to interdisciplinary team members and healthcare consumers.

- Participates with interdisciplinary teams that contribute to role development of faith community nursing practice and faith community advanced practice nursing and wholistic health care.

This appendix is not current and is of historical significance only.

STANDARD 11. COLLABORATION

The faith community nurse collaborates with the patient, spiritual leaders, members of the faith community, and others in the conduct of this specialized nursing practice.

Measurement Criteria:

The faith community nurse:

- Communicates with patient, family, groups, spiritual leaders, and other healthcare providers regarding the care that is needed and the faith community nurse's role in the provision of that care.

- Collaborates in creating a documented plan, focused on outcomes and decisions related to care and delivery of services, that indicates communication and coordination with the patient and others.

- Partners with others to enhance faith-based health care and ultimately care of the patient, through activities such as worship, prayer, education concerning spiritual practices, management of resources, program development, or research opportunities.

- Documents referrals, including provisions for continuity of care outside the faith community.

Additional Measurement Criteria for the Advanced Practice Registered Nurse, Faith Community Nurse:

The advanced practice registered nurse, faith community nurse:

- Partners with other disciplines to enhance faith-based patient care through interdisciplinary activities such as spiritual practices and worship, education, consultation, management, or research opportunities.

- Facilitates an interdisciplinary process with spiritual leaders and other professionals working within the faith community.

- Develops mechanisms to improve communication of plans of care, rationales for plan of care changes, and collaborative discussions to improve patient care.

This appendix is not current and is of historical significance only.

STANDARD 12. ETHICS

The faith community nurse integrates ethical provisions in all areas of practice.

Measurement Criteria:

The faith community nurse:

- Uses *Code of Ethics for Nurses with Interpretive Statements* (ANA 2001) to guide practice.
- Acknowledges and respects tenets of faith and spiritual belief system of a patient.
- Delivers care in a manner that preserves and protects patient autonomy, dignity, rights, and spiritual beliefs and practices.
- Maintains patient confidentiality within religious, legal, and regulatory parameters.
- Serves as a patient advocate assisting patients in developing skills for self-advocacy in support of their spiritual beliefs and practices.
- Maintains a therapeutic and professional patient–nurse relationship within appropriate professional role boundaries.
- Demonstrates a commitment to practicing self-care, growing spiritually, managing stress, and remaining connected both with a centered self and with others.
- Contributes to resolving ethical issues of patients, colleagues, or systems as evidenced in such activities as participating on ethics committees.
- Reports illegal, incompetent, or impaired practices.
- Participates on multidisciplinary and interdisciplinary teams that address ethical risks, benefits, and outcomes.

Additional Measurement Criteria for the Advanced Practice Registered Nurse, Faith Community Nurse:

The advanced practice registered nurse, faith community nurse:

- Informs the patient of the risks, benefits, and outcomes of healthcare regimens.
- Participates on multidisciplinary and interdisciplinary teams that address ethical risks, benefits, and outcomes of programs and decisions that affect health and healthcare delivery.

This appendix is not current and is of historical significance only.

STANDARD 13. RESEARCH

The faith community nurse integrates research findings into practice.

Measurement Criteria:

The faith community nurse:

- Utilizes the best available evidence, including research findings, to guide practice decisions.
- Actively participates in research activities related to spirituality and health at the level appropriate to the faith community nurse's level of education and position. Such activities may include:
  - Identifying clinical and spiritual issues specific to nursing research.
  - Participating in data collection (surveys, pilot projects, formal studies).
  - Participating in a formal research committee or program.
  - Sharing research activities and findings with peers and others.
  - Conducting research.
  - Critically analyzing and interpreting research for application to practice in a faith community.
  - Using research findings in the development of policies, procedures, and standards of practice for wholistic patient care.
  - Incorporating research as a basis for learning.

Additional Measurement Criteria for the Advanced Practice Registered Nurse, Faith Community Nurse:

The advanced practice registered nurse, faith community nurse:

- Contributes to nursing knowledge by conducting or synthesizing research that discovers, examines, and evaluates knowledge, theories, criteria, and creative approaches to integrating spiritual care and nursing care in a faith community.
- Formally disseminates research findings through interdisciplinary activities such as presentations, publications, consultations, and journal clubs.

This appendix is not current and is of historical significance only.

STANDARD 14. RESOURCE UTILIZATION

The faith community nurse considers factors related to safety, effectiveness, cost, and impact on practice in the planning and delivery of nursing services.

Measurement Criteria:

The faith community nurse:

- Evaluates factors such as safety, effectiveness, availability of other resources, cost and benefits, efficiencies, and impact on practice, when choosing between plans of care that would result in the same outcome.
- Assists the patient in identifying and securing appropriate and available resources to address health and spiritually related needs.
- Assigns or delegates tasks, based on the needs and condition of the patient, potential for harm, stability of the patient's condition, complexity of the task, and predictability of the outcome.
- Assists the patient in becoming an informed consumer about the options, costs, risks, and benefits of various interventions.
- Develops innovative solutions and applies strategies to obtain appropriate resources for faith community nursing care.

Additional Measurement Criteria for the Advanced Practice Registered Nurse, Faith Community Nurse:

The advanced practice registered nurse, faith community nurse:

- Utilizes organizational and community resources to formulate multidisciplinary and interdisciplinary plans of care.
- Develops innovative solutions and applies strategies to obtain appropriate resources for patient care problems that address effective resource utilization and maintenance of quality.
- Develops evaluation strategies to demonstrate cost-effectiveness, cost–benefit, and efficiency factors associated with faith community nursing practice.

This appendix is not current and is of historical significance only.

STANDARD 15. LEADERSHIP

The faith community nurse provides leadership in the professional practice setting and the profession.

Measurement Criteria:

The faith community nurse:

- Engages in practice as a recognized member of the staff serving the faith community.

- Works to create and maintain healthy work environments in the local faith community.

- Displays the ability to define a clear vision, the associated goals, and a plan to implement and measure progress towards wholistic health through spiritual care.

- Demonstrates a commitment to continuous, lifelong learning and spiritual growth for self and others.

- Teaches others to succeed by mentoring and other strategies.

- Exhibits creativity and flexibility through times of change.

- Demonstrates energy, excitement, and a passion for quality, spirit-filled work.

- Willingly accepts mistakes by self and others, thereby creating a culture in which risk-taking is not only safe, but expected.

- Inspires loyalty by valuing people as the most precious asset in the faith community.

- Directs the coordination of care within the faith community, across settings, and among caregivers, including training and oversight of unlicensed volunteers in any assigned or delegated tasks.

- Serves in key roles in the faith community by participating on committees, councils, and administrative teams.

- Promotes advancement of faith community nursing and the profession of nursing through participation in professional organizations of nursing and clergy.

This appendix is not current and is of historical significance only.

Additional Measurement Criteria for the Advanced Practice Registered Nurse, Faith Community Nurse:

The advanced practice registered nurse, faith community nurse:

- Works to influence decision-making bodies to recognize spiritual care as integral to improved patient care.

- Designs innovations to effect change in faith community nursing practice and outcomes.

- Provides direction to enhance the creation of multidisciplinary healthcare teams that include providers of spiritual care.

- Initiates revision of protocols or guidelines for outpatient care to reflect evidence-based faith community nursing practice, to reflect the benefit of care management by faith community nurses, or to address emerging problems.

- Promotes communication of information and advancement of faith community nursing through writing, publishing, and presentations for professional or lay audiences.

- Designs innovations to effect change in faith community nursing practice and improve the outcomes of wholistic health and healing.

This appendix is not current and is of historical significance only.

GLOSSARY

Advanced Practice Registered Nurse, Faith Community Nurse (APRN, FCN). An Advanced Practice Registered Nurse, Faith Community Nurse (APRN, FCN) has earned designation as either a clinical nurse specialist or a nurse practitioner, and has also prepared for the role of an FCN. The APRN, FCN builds on the knowledge and skills of a faith community registered nurse by attaining and demonstrating a greater depth and breadth of knowledge, synthesis of data, increased complexity of skills, and interventions in the practice of faith community nursing. (*See also* Faith Community Nurse.)

Assessment. A systematic, dynamic process by which a faith community registered nurse, through interaction with the patient, family, groups, communities, populations, spiritual leaders, and healthcare providers, collects and analyzes data. In addition to spiritual assessment, the faith community registered nurse may include the following dimensions: physical, psychological, sociocultural, cognitive, functional abilities, developmental, economic, environment, and lifestyle.

Caregiver. A person who provides direct care for another, such as a child, dependent adult, the disabled, chronically ill, or spiritually distressed.

Code of ethics. A succinct list of provisions that makes explicit the primary goals, values, and obligations of the profession.

Continuity of care. An interdisciplinary process that includes patients, families, significant others, and appropriate members of a faith community in the development of a coordinated plan of care. This process facilitates the patient's transition between settings and healthcare providers, based on changing needs and available resources.

Criteria. Relevant, measurable indicators of the standards of practice and professional performance. Criteria are revised periodically to remain current with the evolving knowledge and practice of faith community nursing.

Data. Discrete entities that are described objectively without interpretation.

Diagnosis. A clinical judgment about the patient's response to actual, perceived, or potential health concerns or needs. The diagnosis provides the basis for determination of a plan to achieve desired outcomes, establish priorities, and develop a plan of action with the patient. Faith community registered nurses utilize nursing diagnoses or medical diagnoses depending on their education, clinical preparation, and legal authority.

Disease. A biological or psychosocial disorder of structure or function in a patient, especially one that produces specific signs or symptoms or that affects a specific part of the body, mind, or spirit.

This appendix is not current and is of historical significance only.

Documentation. The recording of the assessment, plan of care, interventions, and evaluation of outcomes in a retrievable format that is both confidential and secure for the patient in order to facilitate continuity in meeting desired health outcomes.

Environment. The atmosphere, milieu, or conditions in which an individual lives, works, plays, or carries out their faith practices.

Evaluation. The process of determining the progress toward attainment of expected outcomes and the satisfaction of the patient with those outcomes, for the purpose of modifying the plan. Outcomes include the effectiveness of care, when addressing one's own practice.

Evidence-based practice. A process founded on the collection, interpretation, and integration of valid, important, and applicable patient-reported, clinician-observed, and research-derived evidence. The best available evidence, moderated by patient circumstances and preferences, is applied to improve the quality of clinical judgments.

Faith community. An organization of groups, families, and individuals who share common values, beliefs, religious doctrine, and faith practices that influence their lives, such as a church, synagogue, temple, or mosque, and that functions as a patient system, providing a setting for faith community nursing.

Faith Community Nurse (FCN). A registered professional nurse, actively licensed with the state, who serves as a member of the staff of a faith community. The FCN promotes health as wholeness of the faith community, its groups, families, and individual members, and the community it serves through the practice of nursing as defined by the nurse practice act in the jurisdiction in which the FCN practices and the standards of practice set forth in this document. (*See also* Advanced Practice Registered Nurse, Faith Community Nurse.)

Faith Community Nursing. The specialized practice of professional nursing that focuses on the intentional care of the spirit as part of the process of promoting wholistic health and preventing or minimizing illness in a faith community.

Family. Family of origin or significant others as identified by the patient. The patient may refer to some or all of the members of a faith community as part of their family.

Group. A number of people sharing something in common such as an interest, activity, or spiritual beliefs and practices.

This appendix is not current and is of historical significance only.

Guidelines. Systematic statements that describe recommended actions based on available scientific evidence and expert opinion. Clinical guidelines describe a process of patient care management that has the potential of improving the quality of clinical and consumer decision-making.

Healing. The process of integrating the body, mind, and spirit to bring about wholeness, health, and a sense of spiritual well-being, although the patient's disease may not be cured.

Health. The experience of wholeness, salvation, or shalom. The integration of the spiritual, physical, psychological, and social aspects of the patient to create a sense of harmony with self, others, the environment, and a higher power. Health may be experienced in the presence or absence of disease or injury.

Healthcare providers. Individuals with special expertise who provide healthcare services or assistance to patients. They may include nurses, physicians, spiritual leaders, psychologists, social workers, nutritionists/dietitians, and various therapists.

Health ministry. The promotion of health and healing as part of the mission and service of a faith community to its members and the community it serves.

Health promotion. Activities and interventions that patients undertake to achieve desired health outcomes. Health promotion outcomes may be primary—the prevention of disease and injury; secondary—the early detection and appropriate intervention in illness or brokenness; or tertiary—the promotion of wholeness and sense of well-being when curing may not occur.

Illness. The subjective experience of discomfort, brokenness; the disintegration of body, mind, spirit; disharmony with others, the environment, or a higher power.

Implementation. The carrying out of a plan of action in a spiritual, caring relationship that provides the information, skills, motivation, spiritual or faith tradition rituals, and resources necessary to empower the patient to achieve desired health outcomes.

Interdisciplinary. Reliant on overlapping skills and knowledge of each team member and discipline, resulting in synergistic effects where outcomes are enhanced and more comprehensive than the simple aggregation of any team member's individual efforts.

Multidisciplinary. Reliant on each team member or discipline contributing discipline-specific skills.

This appendix is not current and is of historical significance only.

Patient. Recipient of nursing practice; a human system (faith community, group, family, or individual) and its environment, viewed as an integrated whole for which the Faith Community Nurse provides professional services. The term *patient* is used to provide consistency and brevity, bearing in mind that other terms, such as *client, individual, family, groups, community,* or *population* might be better choices in some instances. When the patient is an individual, the focus is on the health state, problems, or needs of the individual. When the patient is a family or group, the focus is on the health of the unit as a whole or the reciprocal effects of the individual's health on the other members of the unit. When the patient is a community or population, the focus is on personal and environmental health and the health risks of the community or population.

Pastoral care. The practical expression of presence and guidance by a spiritual leader to support, nurture, or encourage the personal, spiritual, and social well-being of an individual or group in the faith community.

Peer review. A collegial, systematic, and periodic process by which Faith Community Nurses are held accountable for their practice and which foster the refinement of one's knowledge, skills, and decision-making.

Plan. A comprehensive outline of the components that need to be completed to attain mutually identified and expected patient outcomes.

Quality of care. The degree to which health services for patients, families, groups, communities, or populations increase the likelihood of desired outcomes, and are consistent with current professional knowledge.

Restorative practices. Nursing interventions that mitigate the impact of illness or disease.

Self-care. Actions a faith community, group, family, or individual take to attain desired wholistic health outcomes when they possess the requisite knowledge, skills, ability, resources, motivation, encouragement, and support.

Spiritual care. Interventions, individual or communal, that facilitate the ability to experience the integration of the body, mind, and spirit to achieve wholeness, health, and a sense of connection to self, others, and a higher power.

Spiritual leader. An individual recognized and authorized by a faith community, such as a clergyperson (pastor, priest, rabbi, shaman), chaplain, or lay minister, who guides and inspires others in the study and nurture of their spiritual beliefs and application of spiritual practices.

This appendix is not current and is of historical significance only.

Standard. An authoritative statement defined and promoted by the profession that reflects the values held by the profession and specialized area of practice, and by which the quality of practice, service, or education can be evaluated.

Supportive practices. Nursing interventions that are oriented toward modification of relationships or the environment to support health.

Well-being. An individual's perception of their own wholistic health.

Wholistic. Based on an understanding that a patient is an interconnected unity and that physical, mental, social, environmental, and spiritual factors need to be included in any interventions. The whole system, whether referring to a human being or a faith community, is greater than the sum of its parts. The preferred term when referring to the type of care provided by a Faith Community Nurse.

This appendix is not current and is of historical significance only.

REFERENCES

American Nurses Association. 2001. *Code of ethics for nurses with interpretive statements.* Washington, DC: Nursebooks.org.

———. 2003. *Nursing's social policy statement.* 2nd edition. Washington, DC: Nursebooks.org.

———. 2004. *Nursing: Scope and standards of practice.* Washington, DC: Nursebooks.org.

Health Ministries Association (HMA) and American Nurses Association (ANA). 1998. *Scope and standards of parish nursing practice.* Washington, DC: American Nurses Publishing.

North American Nursing Diagnosis Association (NANDA). 2005. *Nursing diagnoses: Definitions and classification 2005–2006.* Philadelphia: NANDA International.

Index

P

Parish nurse, 7

Parish nursing, 1, 75

Pastoral Associate, 13, 80

Pastoral care
defined, 110

Patient, 76–77, 80. *See also* Healthcare
consumer
assessment and, 84
collaboration and, 101
consultation, 93
defined, 57, 74, 110
diagnosis and, 85
ethics and, 102
evaluation and, 95
planning and, 88
professional practice evaluation
and, 99
resource utilization and, 104
rights, 102

Peer review/evaluation. *See also*
Collaboration; Communication
defined, 57, 110

Plan
defined, 57, 110

Planning, 72, 80
assessment of, 25
assessment of economic
impact of, 24
collaboration and, 101
collegiality and, 100
competencies for, 24–25
consultation and, 93
coordination of care and, 91
evaluation and, 95
for organizational systems, 25
implementation and,
26–27, 90
leadership and, 105
modification of plan, 25
of practice settings, 24
outcomes identification and, 86
research and, 24
resource utilization and, 104

standard of practice, 24–25, 88–89
strategies for wholeness and
health, 24
strategies for wholistic health, 25

Practice environment, 51, 80. *See also*
Practice settings
collegiality and, 100
communication and, 42
coordination of care and, 91
healthy work environments,
51–52
leadership and, 44, 105
quality of practice and, 41, 97

Practice settings, 14–15, 80

Prescriptive authority and treatment, 72
competencies for, 32
standard of practice, 32, 94

Profession commitment, 15–16

Professional competence in faith
community nursing practice. *See*
Competence

Professional development, 74, 81
collegiality and, 100
education and, 98
leadership and, 105
professional practice evaluation
and, 99
research and, 98

Professional knowledge and faith
community nursing, 17–18

Professional organizations, 105

Professional practice evaluation, 73
collegiality and, 100
competencies for, 47–48
health teaching and health
promotion, 92
standard of professional performance,
47–48, 99

Q

Quality of care, 79
defined, 57, 110

Quality of life, 82, 87